SCLERODERMA

A New Role For

Patients and Families

Michael Brown

Scleroderma Press
Los Angeles

1st ed.
Includes references, footnotes

ISBN 0-9717524-0-0
Library of Congress Control Number: 2002090223

SCLERODERMA: A New Role For Patients and Families

Index
Scleroderma (disease), Chronic Illness, Caregiving, Self-help, Medical, Health

Edited by Richard C. Williams

Book cover design by Todd E. Weiner

Other scleroderma related books by Scleroderma Press
PMO: Personal Medical Organizer
For Scleroderma Patients

Printed and bound in the United States of America

Dedicated to

scleroderma patients
and their families

CONTENTS

Foreword

To most of the populace the word "scleroderma" has no meaning. When they first hear the word, they often respond with, "What is that again?" Those of you who are reading this book know all too well what *scleroderma* is. Fortunately the majority of people who have scleroderma will be able to adapt to its symptoms and limitations.

For an unfortunate few, scleroderma can be a catastrophe, which causes great suffering, marked limitation of function, severe involvement of the internal organs—and death. This type of rapid progression (which is fortunately unusual) was documented in the made-for-television movie, "For Hope," directed by Bob Saget. "For Hope" documented the case of Bob's sister and of the meshagass that surrounded the family, all of whom were ill prepared to deal with this kind of catastrophe. Saget's motives for making the movie were partly to raise the public awareness about scleroderma but also to provide him with a catharsis for the grief that he felt about his sister's loss.

Presently there are textbooks to teach physicians and healthcare professionals about scleroderma. For patients and families, *The Scleroderma Book* was written in "lay-speak" by Maureen Mayes, MD, MPH. It addresses in plain English many of the physical, functional and emotional issues that face patients with scleroderma and their loved ones.

Until now, there hasn't been a book that addresses the *non-medical* issues from the perspective of patients and families; this book does. It was written by Mike Brown, a man, like Bob Saget, who suffered through a difficult case of scleroderma—only in this instance he was the caregiver to his wife.

The book's purpose is three-fold. The first purpose is to advise patients and their families to become proactive and to participate in making medical decisions. Secondly, it is to inform patients about issues that have not been discussed elsewhere. The third provides him catharsis: in this instance the catharsis is channeled into a book designed to provide tools for empowering scleroderma patients and their families.

Mike's book addresses issues such as: finding sources of reliable information about scleroderma, picking a caring and knowledgeable physician, interacting with healthcare providers, finding insurance and financial aid, caregiving—and a host of other everyday, nitty-gritty issues that surround the care of anyone with a chronic illness like scleroderma. This book contains little pearls of wisdom that can benefit anyone with scleroderma, including those who have the mildest case of the disease.

One of the book's objectives is to have patients and families "get involved and be proactive." Physicians frequently find it difficult to "take care" of people who do not themselves become involved in their own care. Many of us see our role, not as servants, but as teachers, to help patients learn more about their disease so that they can better take care of themselves. I agree with Mike that it is absolutely essential for improving treatment outcomes to have patients and their families actively involved in decision making and being proactive in their own care.

The second objective is to direct patients and their families to resources that they may need but may not know about. The book explores several of these resources in detail: how to navigate the Internet to get the most out of it without getting confused by all the misinformation and hype; how to find a physician who "fits your style" and is knowledgeable about scleroderma; how to interact with healthcare providers and physicians to get the most out of each visit; how and where to look for insurance; finding options and resources to help a family's financial situation if they lose the ability to work; finding organizations that can help them physically and functionally to improve their life.

The third objective is catharsis—but he does it with a twist. He weaves a story about what it took to care for and nurture his gravely ill wife. The twist: he reflects on his role as caregiver and finally on his role as emotional support and soul mate for his wife. He lets the reader see the problems of caregiving—and hopefully that will help improve the lot of caregiver and of care receiver alike. The story concludes with what probably is the most important part of caring—the role in which both caregiver and care receiver take and receive nourishment—building an emotional bond that ultimately improves the quality of life.

March 1, 2002

Dr. Philip J. Clements, MD, MPH
President, Scleroderma
Clinical Trials Consortium
Professor of Medicine
UCLA School of Medicine

Acknowledgements

I wish my family had been as lucky as most other Americans and never heard of scleroderma—that's what we all would have liked. Some of us have learned a lot about scleroderma, others know less; but one thing is for sure, whatever any of us have learned, it was probably learned the hard way. Motivation to write this book was due in large part by my frustration of knowing that scleroderma patients and families continuously struggle to learn what others already know.

Before I even began writing, I knew that aside from personal experience, my approach to this book would be heavily influenced by the kind of person I am. Being a self-professed "information junky" by nature and part market researcher by trade is fundamental to how this book is presented. Research is not a one-person effort. I am smart enough to know (and accept) what I don't know. As a result, I depended a great deal upon people whose experience and expertise exceeded mine.

I was extremely fortunate to have the help of Tallien Perry in sorting out many of the legal and insurance issues. As a healthcare attorney, former editor-in-chief of the California Health Law News, and friend, she dedicated many hours to reviewing not only the technical points, but the entire manuscript.

Scleroderma means living in a world of uncertainty and anxiety. As a leading investigator in scleroderma research, the involvement of Dr. Phil Clements has been a source of comfort for many of us over the years. It is with gratitude, not only for the foreword he provided for this book, but most important, for his personal and professional commitment to fighting this disease, that I thank him for his dedication.

I also called upon many people within the scleroderma community. Besides the input of dozens of patients and advocates, I also received invaluable comments from scleroderma organizations.

My thanks goes to the Scleroderma Foundation for its helpful feedback, and especially to CEO, Peter Giusti, whose leadership I have always respected for keeping the focus on the patient; Carolyn Weller, RN, National Director of Education, whose insights reflect the pulse of the patient; and Tim Hanke, National Director of Publications and Internet Services, for his dogged determination in getting the SF message out.

In addition to depending upon research and feedback, my own personal experience with healthcare professionals had an impact on the tone of this book; generally, it was a very good experience. A positive experience with the healthcare system these days can only be the result of coming into contact with many good people. But, it goes beyond credit and gratitude that I single-out the personal and professional dedication of our primary care physician, Dr. Dennis Lewis, of the UCLA Medical Center. He was not only the right doctor for us; he was also the best.

On a personal note, one of the nicer aspects of publishing this book was having the eager support of family and friends. Especially gratifying was the work provided by Todd Weiner, graphic artist, who designed the cover; and Rick Williams, English instructor, Rogue College, Oregon, for the editing. In addition, my thanks to Kalman Winnick and Lydia Weisman, both an invaluable source of caring support.

To be the best I can, I need balance in my life. Synchronizing all of my priorities, such as family, work, and dreams, gives me that balance. But I know that without having family as the *centerpiece* of my priorities, everything else becomes irrelevant.

Fortunately, my three daughters, Hillary, Lauren, and Devin are my centerpiece. They have spoiled me with their love, support and confidence (more than I deserve), and have made it possible for me to appreciate and enjoy life. I love you guys.

March 1, 2002   Michael Brown

In memory of

Karen Brown

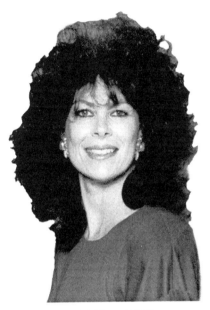

1950 – 2000

Introduction

BACKGROUND

Karen was my wife for over thirty years. Although some of her experiences as a scleroderma patient are used anecdotally throughout this book, they are only for the purpose of illustrating particular points.

It is not wise to compare medical conditions from one scleroderma patient to the next. The very nature of scleroderma makes it impossible to use a single medical case to describe the disease. Each patient is like a snowflake, with no two being exactly alike. No book I've ever read has been able to portray the disease so that patients can specifically relate it to their own case. This book doesn't even try.

Although Karen had many medical *involvements* that were similar to other scleroderma patients, it needs to be noted that, because of the number of ways the disease attacked, and the speed and severity of its progression, she was the rarest of exceptions, even for a disease that is defined by exceptions.

Within the first six months of diagnosis, she went through excruciating pain; she was using a cane to walk within three months, a walker by the fifth month, and confined to a wheelchair by the sixth month. Within the next four months, she experienced congestive heart failure and a 60 percent loss of lung function. She was unable to eat and received nutrition through an IV, and she became permanently dependent upon kidney dialysis.

I was initially hesitant to use specific examples of Karen's case in writing this book. I was afraid that it might unnecessarily scare some patients (especially the newly diagnosed)—and that would have defeated the purpose of this book. I hope that Dr. Clement's foreword put any unnecessary fears to rest.

But beyond the medical issues, which cannot be compared, the non-medical issues that Karen faced are remarkably similar to what other scleroderma patients encounter. Regardless of whether someone has a mild case or more severe form of the disease, the issues presented in this book, such as finding a doctor, insurance, alternative medicine, family and caregiving—are very similar for everyone.

WHY THIS BOOK WAS WRITTEN

I wish this book didn't have to be written, or, that there would be nobody to read it. From personal experience, though, I know that, despite the growing amount of information available for scleroderma patients, it's not always easy to find what they need, when they need it. This book was written because it is the book that I wanted, but couldn't find, when Karen was diagnosed with scleroderma in 1998.

Without easily accessible information, Karen and I educated ourselves pretty much the same way as other scleroderma patients and families—and it was all the hard way. This book was written so that you can reduce the time and effort needed to be informed and get on with what truly matters: making the most of your medical choices.

From the beginning, Karen and I knew that there was no gold standard for the treatment of scleroderma, and not a cure in sight. But for us, the worst part of the disease was our inability to get our questions answered. We didn't want to be bystanders and leave all the decisions to the impersonal bureaucracy of managed care. We wanted to be a part of the decision making process and were unwilling to passively accept what we got.

Scleroderma requires an overwhelming and instant need for information and experience. Trying to understand and navigate the intricacies of all the issues is a forbidding task under the best of circumstances. Doing it during a medical crisis is almost impossible. I tried my best, researching thousands of hours, trying to find answers to the *crises of the day* and maybe even a cure along the way.

I researched libraries, database information services, public and private organizations, and the Internet. Most of the time the information helped, but, by the end of the day, I usually ended up richer in data than in answers. From the first day of diagnosis, until her death in 2000, there was simply never enough time to figure out what we should do or even how to best use the information we found.

When it was over, I had thousands of hours of experience and countless pieces of paper and megabytes of information. Looking over it after she was gone, I was overwhelmed and shocked to see how much material I had collected. Much of it I never used because it was either in a disorganized state or forgotten about.

Our battle was lost and scleroderma no longer controls every minute of my family's life. But it is not completely in the past for me either. I think about the other battles that were lost before Karen. And I think about the many patients who do survive their own battles by keeping informed, by finding emotional strength, and sometimes by being just plain lucky.

Today the disease continues—not only in the United States, but all around the world. There are scores of newly diagnosed patients starting this vicious cycle every day. Some will have an easier time, others worse. But they will all have to endure this same merciless process of not knowing anything at first, and thereafter, never being able to catch up with all that they need to know—just like Karen, just like the countless numbers before her.

It's this perpetual and senseless cycle that has kept me involved. Otherwise, it would have been easy to throw away all the material and experience I collected and wash away the memories of the suffering. But seeing scleroderma first-hand was the cruelest thing I have ever witnessed, and I choose not to forget.

Everybody has a contribution to make that can help others. Everybody has experience that can shorten the learning curve for others. You don't need to make all the same mistakes that others have already made. You don't need to go down all the same dead-ends. You don't need to learn on your own what others already know. The essence of the experience and information I have is in this book. This is my contribution.

PURPOSE OF THIS BOOK

Over the years there have been many advances in research and therapies. We are now much closer to finding the answers we need; even so, there is still no cure. This fact leaves many patients feeling helpless and fatalistic, reducing them to mere spectators to their own disease.

Rather than sitting on the sidelines, this book helps define a new role for you, the patient, and your family. This new role is designed to empower you as a self-directed patient. It is based upon understanding the issues and determining what's right for you, so that you can chart your own course and become a full partner in your own care. Self-directed patients tend to make more accurate observations of their own condition, ask well-focused questions, and are better prepared to make the best of their medical choices.

This book does not replace a doctor (or any other professional for that matter). It doesn't offer any medical opinions either. Medical and other professional advice should be left to the experts.

I am not a doctor, but a searcher that spent a 1,000 days as a 24-hour-a-day caregiver and advocate managing Karen's care. The basic concepts in this book are not new. A self-directed patient is responsible and involved in his or her own medical care; this trend has already permeated and affected many aspects of medical care. What this book does do is to present these concepts so that each scleroderma patient can apply them to their own needs.

This book is a guide and resource to the many issues scleroderma presents, so you can be informed and make the most of your choices. Not all self-directed patients are the same; it is up to each one to define the level of responsibility and involvement they want.

This new role is ideally suited for scleroderma patients because it lets them zero-in on the individual care needed for this extraordinarily individualized disease. Addressing your specific needs can have dramatic benefits. That is what this book is all about. But this concept may not appeal to everyone.

For those that think they are not capable of effectively dealing with all of the issues, I believe that they will find that this book is laid out in such a way as to maximize its usefulness for each individual. For those that have complete trust and confidence in their doctor and don't feel it's the role of the patient to be this involved, this book may have limited appeal.

Regardless of the level of involvement you choose, you need to do your homework, and the best place to start is learning the basics about the disease. Within a year of Karen's diagnosis, I considered myself very knowledgeable about scleroderma. Yet when Dr. Maureen Mayes' book, *Scleroderma: A Guide for Patients and Families*[1] was published in 1999, I still found it very helpful, particularly in putting all the various aspects of the disease into perspective. You need to understand the medical issues as well as the issues covered in this book. Dr. Mayes' book is a good starting place for everyone.

Some have become *patient-experts* on the disease and have even read medical books that are intended for doctors and other medical professionals.[2] These people probably know more about how the disease affects their specific case than many doctors do. This level of involvement doesn't work for everyone, nor will it result in getting them a medical degree, but it does put them in an excellent position to maximize their care.

This book has many benefits, but unfortunately, it doesn't suggest a cure or have all the answers. Then again, neither do your doctors. By becoming a full partner in your own care, you can help yourself, and even make your own contribution by sharing your benefits with your doctors and other patients.

Before scleroderma, many families spent a good deal of time trying to provide a measure of control and security in their lives. Scleroderma takes much of that away. Scleroderma goes beyond the viciousness of many other diseases because of its unpredictability. There are many diseases that can debilitate or kill. But scleroderma stands apart, not only in the variety of ways it can do its damage, but also in the indiscriminate way it strikes. The number of ways it can attack is only limited by the number of its victims. It can leave patients feeling hopeless and helpless, just when it is most important for them to take control.

Some may embrace every aspect of this book. Certain parts may not apply to you. Others may use it as a resource as specific issues come up. It is your life and your right to be as involved as you want. This book is your tool, but the choice of how you use it is up to you.

Chapter 1

Scleroderma Update

We know much more about scleroderma now than we did twenty years ago. It's a source of hope as we continuously find new pieces to this puzzle and are thus better able to educate ourselves as well as the general public. The increase in our understanding of this disease has been especially encouraging during the last three to five years, because the rate of progress, on all fronts, seems to be accelerating.

The ones who are perhaps best able to appreciate this progress are scleroderma patients who were diagnosed many years ago. They have had years to absorb the constant flow of information and to interact with other patients.

For newly diagnosed patients, the progress may be more difficult to appreciate. A new patient is more likely to see how much more needs to be done than what's been accomplished. In addition, many new patients tend to be isolated, either by lack of information, or by the depression and denial that often accompanies their sudden status as scleroderma patients.

Public Awareness

In the past, hardly anybody knew what scleroderma was; but that is now changing. As it does, scleroderma patients have had some of the burden of feeling *alone* lifted as others have become more aware of the disease. Public awareness has also helped put the disease on the map enough to increase research funding.

Some of the success in public awareness is a result of the involvement of personalities, like Bob Saget and Jason Alexander. Both got involved because the disease struck close family members. Others, such as Darrell Gilbert, an Oklahoma State Representative, whose wife Kathy has scleroderma, used his political position by urging his fellow lawmakers to authorize a Scleroderma Awareness Day.[3]

The few public figures that have gotten involved have had a substantial impact. At the same time, the ranks of everyday people spreading the word have also swelled. It's been a word-of-mouth effort for most, with others actively getting the message to the media. A database search of recent stories in newspapers across the country came up with over four hundred articles that profiled scleroderma patients, treatments, and support groups; that's not including the exposure on radio, television, and in other media.

Along with greater public awareness has also come an increase in contradictory and misleading information. Misinformation dilutes the value of the accurate information the public receives. Even doctors sometimes seem to have trouble getting their facts right. As an example, one doctor, who has a syndicated health advisory column, suggested that a scleroderma patient look into Relaxin because it was showing a lot of "promise."[4] This was four months after the manufacturer, Connetics Corporation, abandoned its Relaxin clinical trial due to poor results. It must have been very disheartening for the reader to be led to another dead-end, especially by a doctor.

How Many Have Scleroderma?

One area of confusion is the discrepancy in the number of people reported by the media to have the disease. The count depends upon whom you ask. Nobody seems to figure the same way. The most generally accepted number at this time is that 300,000 Americans have scleroderma. That would calculate to just over 1,000 people with scleroderma for every one million of the population. This number includes all forms of the disease, and is assumed to apply worldwide.

Some say it is a rare disease, others say its numbers exceed those of other well-known diseases. Here are some recent numbers from the media:

Kansas City Star, Jul 17, 1999
"It affects 150,000 people in the United States..."

Times - Picayune; New Orleans, La.; Jun 25, 2000.
"Scleroderma afflicts about 700,000 people in the United States."

New York Times Jul 4, 2000
"An estimated 75,000 to 100,000 Americans, mostly women of childbearing age, suffer from scleroderma."

Daily Telegraph, UK- Feb 6, 2001
"Some 4,000 people in Britain are affected by scleroderma..." Based on the total population of Britain, this figure should be many times higher if the incidence of scleroderma is roughly the same throughout the world.

On the other side of this issue are the drug companies. They tend to sometimes be lower in their estimates of the number of people with scleroderma. This might have something to do with their desire to get the FDA to designate their potential product as an orphan[5] drug. The orphan drug designation applies to diseases that affect fewer than 200,000 people. If qualified, the drug company is eligible for tax credits and extended time to exclusively market the product without competition. It can also be said that drug companies can float lower patient numbers by counting only the number of scleroderma patients with a specific involvement that pertains to their drug.

What do all these numbers mean? They mean that the figures quoted in the media are creating some confusion with the public, which adds to the problem of providing an accurate image of the disease. "Estimates for the number of people in the United States with systemic sclerosis, according to the National Institute of Health (NIH), range from 40,000 to 165,000. By contrast, a survey that included all scleroderma-related disorders, including Raynaud's Phenomenon, suggested a number between 250,000 and 992,500."[6]

Not having an accurate count and a consistent image of scleroderma is a huge barrier in fighting this disease. It will likely become a greater issue in the future as the media spotlight on the disease increases. In the past, different numbers cited in various news stories weren't obvious to a general population that was still unaware of the disease. But now, many of the advocacy and public awareness programs are becoming more effective. Being in sync, not only in quoting the number of patients, but also in portraying a consistent image of the disease that the public can understand, is becoming much more important. With so many faces to the disease, it's not an easy task.

The Importance of the Scleroderma Registry

Another side of the issue goes well beyond just determining the number of people with scleroderma. It has to do with obtaining individual patient profiles and putting them into a database with thousands of other patient profiles. The collection and analysis of this information is referred to as the disease's epidemiology. It can provide insights and possible patterns in the occurrence of the disease. It helps to determine if there are any social, geographic, occupational, or environmental factors that contribute to the disease. It never identifies a specific patient's name, address, phone number, social security number, or even age, unless the patient specifically authorizes the release of such information for research or other specific purposes.

The National Institute of Arthritis and Musculoskeletal and Skin Diseases (NIAMS)[7] has taken a major step in studying the epidemiology of scleroderma. A press release dated June 2001, announced the creation of the National Scleroderma Registry. "Its overall objective is to identify genes that influence susceptibility to scleroderma . . ."

The registry will study families with only one case of scleroderma and those with more than one case (known as multiplex families). Specifically, the registry will:

- Determine the frequency with which scleroderma occurs in more than one family member and how often other autoimmune diseases (such as lupus) occur in families with at least one case of scleroderma.

- Conduct a nationwide search to identify and enroll multiplex families.

- Collect and store genetic material (DNA) and blood serum from scleroderma patients and from friends and in-laws as unrelated controls.

11

- Collaborate with scientists at the University of Texas, Houston, to identify susceptible genes for scleroderma.

- Advertise the availability of the DNA repository as a resource to scientists studying genes associated with scleroderma and other autoimmune diseases.

Although a milestone, the success of this program will depend, in large part, on scleroderma patients stepping forward and identifying themselves so they can be included in the registry. It is vitally important that every scleroderma patient contact the registry to be included.[8]

Can't Prove It, Can't Disprove It

When diagnosed with scleroderma, a lot of people think, "this wasn't supposed to happen to me!" Scleroderma doesn't fit with what anybody thought that life had in store for them. Many look for reasons as to how they "got" scleroderma. Environmental factors almost always seem to be at the top of the list. And there seems to be good reason for this suspicion. But at this time, there is only the presence of environmental "suspects" that might possibly "trigger" this disease and the likelihood that some people are "genetically predisposed" to the disease.

For now though, nothing has been proven, and, unfortunately, not very much has been disproved either. Not knowing can be emotionally debilitating; it breeds fear and depression: hardly the ingredients necessary to fight the disease.

A year before Karen was diagnosed with scleroderma, we moved into a new house. Not long after the move, our dog, Gizmo, died of some mysterious viral or bacterial infection. Several months later when Karen was diagnosed with scleroderma, friends started to talk about some connection between the two, implying that there must be "something in the house." Throughout the course of Karen's disease, the "Gizmo Factor" (as it came to be known) was not only emotionally debilitating, it haunted her. There were even a couple of friends that were more than a little uncomfortable in stepping foot inside our house, even for a brief visit.

During her illness, doctors discouraged me from having the house tested for any of these "environmental suspects." Just for the sake of "knowing," after her death, I again pursued the idea of having the house tested. I got a referral from an occupational medical specialist. He referred me to an industrial hygienist. I was told it was a needle in a haystack. Unless I could tell the hygienist what to look for, it was useless. It seemed ludicrous for me to tell the hygienist what to look for, and no one would give me any advise. Even if someone had told me what to look for, the chances of proving a link to scleroderma were practically nil. It was basically an open-ended pursuit, which would only conclude when I ran out of money; and it still wouldn't prove anything for sure. Even though I desperately wanted "answers," I chose to do nothing.

It is not unusual for a scleroderma patient to suspect an environmental culprit:

The Daily Telegraph; London (UK); Feb 6, 2001.
An airline worker believes "a concentration of airport chemicals combined with whiplash from a car accident might have provoked scleroderma."

Puget Sound News; Nov 7, 2000
Scleroderma victim thinks a nearby crematorium caused it.

Controversy has surrounded claims by some patients that leaks from silicone breast implants caused their arthritis, as well other disorders such as scleroderma. The manufacturer, Dow Corning, funded a study that they claimed conclusively proved that their product had nothing to do with the women's disease. The women were unconvinced—claiming that Dow Corning paid for the answer they wanted, thus proving nothing.

Chapter 1

Scleroderma Research

One of the most difficult aspects to understand about scleroderma is that it is not a single disease. "Scleroderma is really a symptom of a group of diseases."[9] Most diseases have one or two components. Scleroderma has at least four. It is an autoimmune disease; it affects the vascular system, creates fibrosis in tissue, and is also an inflammatory disease. This is why scleroderma is so complicated.

As anyone knows who has ever seen a group of scleroderma patients, they all look different. From the localized forms of Morphea and Linear Scleroderma, to patients with systemic forms, they not only look different, but the requirements of their medical care can also be quite different. For some patients, the affects of the disease are visually obvious. For others, the disease isn't just skin-deep, and affects the muscles, joints, and internal organs.

The seemingly limitless ways for these four components to interact makes it all the more difficult for researchers. As a result, investigators have tended to take one of two approaches in their hunt for answers: one is to carry out basic research, often at the cellular level, to try and understand the cause and determine possible treatments that might lead to a cure.

The other path tries to develop therapies that contain the disease, or treat specific symptoms, in the hope of prolonging the quality of life of patients. These therapies are not cures but are more likely to produce treatments for specific "involvements," such as lungs, heart, gastro-intestinal, and kidneys.

Research Funding

No one will disagree that scleroderma research is grossly under-funded, in spite of the fact that the investment in research dollars has been growing at a double-digit rate for several years now. Yet it is still inadequate, because the amount of these increases are based upon the miniscule dollars allocated five and ten years ago.

But what is considered miniscule can be a matter of opinion. In a newspaper article in the UK's *Daily Telegraph, Feb 6, 2001*, a scleroderma authority was quoted as saying that they wished they had as much funding as the U.S. " ...in the United States the disease attracts sizeable research funding. Here, however, it has been regarded as an orphan disease." Sad to say, while scleroderma research funding in the U.S. is inadequate, that so many other countries are so much worse off.

Government Funding

Government funding for scleroderma research has been on the upswing. Compared to the amount of money allocated a few years ago, it could even be said to be generous. But another way of looking at it is to compare the current research dollars spent to what scleroderma costs society. What does it cost society? There is no exact answer, but examples of some of the costs include lost job productivity, cost of disability, and astronomical healthcare bills that end up increasing everyone else's health insurance premium. If an estimate had to be made, then $100 million per year would be very conservative. Compared to the single digit millions now spent on research, it wouldn't seem difficult to justify a ten or even twenty fold increase of current funding. And, that of course, doesn't even take into consideration the most important cost of all: the personal toll on patients and families.

Private Funding

Nonprofit charities make a substantial contribution to scleroderma research. They have been able to increase the amount of money raised for research and are producing a louder, more focused awareness campaign that provides the public, business, and government with a clearer understanding of the disease and the need for more research.

Until recently, there were three major scleroderma organizations; The United Scleroderma Foundation, The Scleroderma Federation, and The Scleroderma Research Foundation[10](SRF). In the late 1990's, some hoped that all three would come together as one organization. As it turned out, the first two did join together, forming the Scleroderma Foundation[11](SF).

Some people within the scleroderma community are disappointed that there are still two organizations. To them, one organization would eliminate the duplication of expense and effort and would provide a much stronger voice on behalf of all scleroderma patients in the areas of research, patient support, and public awareness.

On the other hand, others felt that with so much more to know and understand about the disease, a multi-pronged approach also makes sense. Their thinking was based upon the fact that without a proven theory, different perspectives and approaches improves the chances of finding answers.

Although there is always a risk that research projects conducted by multiple organizations might duplicate one another, publishing results in peer reviewed medical journals allow all members of the scleroderma scientific community to share their findings. Some investigators are even involved in projects of multiple organizations, including the National Institute of Health (NIH). This helps keep scientists better informed and reduces the chance of duplication, and sometimes even encourages an opportunity for cross-institutional collaboration.

Some people feel that only the federal government has the money to make a big impact on scleroderma research, but scleroderma organizations have also played a crucial role. Not only have they provided valuable input regarding the direction of government research, they often are ahead of government research in exploring new areas.

Identifying new areas to delve into has sometimes made scleroderma organizations an incubator and source of seed money for innovative research. If the organization's investigation proves itself, the government can continue the funding. This was the case with an SRF funded investigation on Raynaud's Phenomenon in 2000, and also with a recent SF supported trial of oral type I collagen.

The primary difference between the SRF and the SF is in their approach to research. The SF utilizes the same traditional methods to review and evaluate research as the NIH. In contrast, the SRF funds their own cross-functional team of researchers from the medical, academic and public-private sectors. The SRF believes that it can shorten the time in finding a cure by having their investigators share their findings with each other immediately, rather than waiting for publication and review.

A key difference between the two organizations is that the SRF is focused only on research that might lead to a cure and the SF funds research for both treatments as well as research that might lead to a cure. In addition to research, the SF is the only organization that has nationwide patient support groups and also provides educational literature for both patients and doctors. Each organization has a separate public awareness campaign.

The Consolidation of Research

As research dollars for scleroderma continues to expand, so do the number of places that researchers look for answers. This fact becomes obvious when searching the CRISP database (Computer Retrieval of Information on Scientific Projects),[12] which tracks federally funded biomedical research projects that are conducted at universities, hospitals, and other research institutions. Although it is not the ultimate word on the status of scleroderma research, it is very reveling. In the early 1990s, there was never more than twenty scleroderma research projects funded in a given year. By the late 1990s, government funded scleroderma projects had increased to an average of about one hundred per year.

The expansion of research is also behind a move toward more consolidation and collaboration. Universities, drug companies, government and private organizations are slowly coming together, pooling their resources and "cross pollinating." It is hoped that this will lead to opportunities for them to learn from each other, and speed the research process.

Working closer together is also due, in part, to the very nature of scleroderma; although the causes may be different, many of the secondary involvements associated with scleroderma are similar to other diseases. Examples are: lung disease, pulmonary hypertension, and GI diseases. So it would make sense, as an example, that an investigation primarily funded through a lung disease research organization might also have the support of scleroderma investigators. The result of this can be seen on the next few pages; there are several new drug therapies listed that were primarily developed for another disease, but have also proven beneficial for scleroderma patients.

The Scleroderma Clinical Trials Consortium (SCTC)[13] is an organization that is helping to bring independent researchers together. It has over fifty centers to conduct trials by a well-organized group of researchers who are experienced in scleroderma.

This organization has been growing in prominence lately. It is currently in the process of expanding its alliances with both private and government organizations, and, as a tax-exempt entity, also seeks private support.

There has recently been a greater effort to expand the SCTC internationally, but apparently there is some reluctance. One of the delays is due to the time it takes to gain trust among international researchers so that they can work effectively together.

The government is also trying to consolidate research among related diseases.[14] In September 2000,

Congress signed legislation[15] that created a permanent Autoimmune Disease Coordinating Committee[16] within the NIH.[17] It will coordinate all autoimmune research activities throughout federal agencies, including the Centers for Disease Control and Prevention (CDC)[18] and the Food and Drug Administration (FDA).[19]

This new category of research will have the clout of 50 million people instead of scleroderma's 300,000. Specifically, it will be the task of the Autoimmune Disease Coordinating Committee to provide a broad range of research studies relating to biomedical, psychosocial, and rehabilitative issues, including basic research to determine causes of the diseases and studies that address their frequency. It is still too early to tell, but hopefully this will translate into new funding opportunities.

"Measuring" Scleroderma

Scleroderma is a disease that is very difficult to measure. This is especially true when trying to determine if a new treatment works. Of course, there are baseline tests that measure specific organs, such as lungs and kidney function. But for those treatments and clinical trials where the expectation is for overall improvement of a patient's condition, it has been difficult to gauge. Researchers worldwide are continuously trying to establish what is called "standard outcome measures" for clinical trials so that results can be compared over time and to different patient groups.

Developing a standard method to evaluate the severity and progression of scleroderma has also been very challenging for investigators. One current method is to measure the thickness of skin for those patients with both skin and internal involvement. The thinking goes that if the skin thickens, it is presumed that the disease is worsening internally as well. If the skin "softens" and becomes thinner, then it is an indication that the internal involvement has also improved.

The most common way to measure skin thickness is through a "skin pinch" test, where the doctor lightly pinches seventeen points on the body and rates the thickness of the skin on a scale of zero to three, three being the thickest. Sometimes this is referred to in clinical trials that specify a particular range of skin scores for patients to be eligible. But this test is somewhat subjective, because it is done manually, and can vary greatly if the patient is retaining more fluids than usual, or is on kidney dialysis.

High tech solutions that measure the condition of the skin are underway. From Sweden, there is an effort to develop a skin score that is based on an ultrasound. Here in the U.S., another method is being developed that measures the skin with a laser beam that can examine the biomechanical properties of the skin.

Going beyond just measuring the skin, a wider-based scale that rates the severity of individual areas of involvement, such as vascular, skin, joints, muscle, and individual organs, is being developed. This will allow "groups of patients participating in multicenter trials and reported in the literature to be directly compared and will permit longitudinal evaluation of the course of disease in both individual patients and groups."[20]

Government Sponsored Research

Government research for scleroderma is primarily funded through NIAMS, which is part of the NIH. Much of its research efforts on scleroderma are conducted at the Specialized Center of Research (SCOR)[21] located at the University of Texas-Houston.

Past and present research sponsored by the NIH and other organizations has led to a better understanding and treatments of the disease in the following areas:[22]

- Gene Research
  Research on the Oklahoma Choctaw Native Americans, a group that has a very high rate of

scleroderma, has led to identification of a gene that is associated with scleroderma. It is hoped that these findings might enable doctors to identify people that have a genetically higher risk of the disease.

- Immune system changes (and particularly how those changes affect the lungs) in early diffuse systemic sclerosis.

- The role of blood vessel malfunction, cell death, and autoimmunity in scleroderma.

- Skin changes in laboratory mice in which a genetic defect prevents the breakdown of collagen, leading to thick skin and patchy hair loss. Scientists hope that by studying these mice, they can answer many questions about skin changes in scleroderma.

- The study of tiny blood vessels of people with scleroderma. By studying these changes, scientists hope to find the cause of cold sensitivity in Raynaud's phenomenon and how to control the problem.

Private Research

- **Fetal Cell Research**

Making headlines out of preliminary and incomplete research does little to help scleroderma patients, but it does sell news. This has been the case regarding fetal cell research and scleroderma. One headline in The Times, London (UK), on Feb 19, 2001, read, "Babies' tissue may be killing mothers." Many other papers around the world echoed similar themes.

There has been no conclusion reached yet as to the role, if any, that fetal cells play in scleroderma. What researchers have found though, is that during pregnancy, the mother and the fetus literally exchange cells, leaving identifiable fetal cells inside the mother after birth. Some researchers believe lingering fetal cells may contribute to autoimmune diseases by interfering with the mother's immune system. This might help explain why scleroderma strikes four times as many women than men.

This fetal cell exchange is like a mini-gene transfer between mother and fetus. Hong Kong researchers have found that fetal DNA accounts for about 3 percent of the total in a pregnant woman.[23] It has been suggested that some of these cells can remain active for decades in the mother and can later interfere with the mother's immune system and trigger scleroderma.

Another clue in this on-going puzzle came from a mouse. Retired breeding mice that had produced scores of litters were induced with a scleroderma-like disease by injecting vinyl chloride, a material found in many plastic products and implicated in human scleroderma. In the injected mice, the number of fetal cells detected in the blood increased fifty-fold. The research suggested that fetal cells might combine with environmental factors to cause scleroderma.

Even though fetal cell research is providing valuable clues, it is still only a piece of the puzzle. It does little to explain why women that have never been pregnant, or men for that matter, get the disease.

Stem Cell Transplants

Stem Cell Transplants for scleroderma patients is in its early stages. It shows promise but is still a very dangerous procedure. It is only for the worst cases at this time. In the initial study, a combination of radiation and cancer drugs were used to kill the immune system of the patient. The patient then received back his or her own transplanted stem cells that were extracted before the treatment. This allows these new stem cells to grow into bone marrow. The result is that the patient gets a new immune system—hopefully one that won't continue to overproduce collagen.

The Phase I/II Trial Impact Report[24] provided results from forty-one patients. Sixty-nine percent of the patients improved their skin score by greater than 25 percent, 7 percent deteriorated. In the past, the mortality rate has been as high as 25 percent. It is expected that, in the future, a 10 percent mortality factor related to this procedure should be anticipated.

Drug Therapies

ACE Inhibitors (angiotensin converting enzyme)

The use of ACE inhibitors has greatly reduced the affects of kidney involvement in scleroderma patients. There is evidence that the use of ACE inhibitors can actually heal the kidneys of people on dialysis for scleroderma-related kidney failure. As many as half of the people who continue ACE inhibitors while on dialysis may be able to go off dialysis in twelve to eighteen months.

Flolan® (Epoprostenol)

For some patients, the intravenous drug Flolan can be a very effective treatment for pulmonary hypertension. It tends to open blood vessels, thereby increasing capacity for exercise and has even reduced a number of fingertip ulcers. Long term side affects have not yet been determined, and abrupt withdrawal or interruption of treatment is very dangerous.

Tracleer® (Bosentan)

Tracleer is one of the newest drugs for pulmonary hypertension. Orphan drug status put this oral treatment on the fast tract, and was approved by the FDA in December 2001. The drug treats the disease by reducing the amount of a substance called endothelin in blood vessels. Like many new promising drugs, there is a need for caution: clinical trials indicated about 11 percent of patients experienced abnormal but reversible liver enzyme elevations and a risk of birth defects. Patients need to undergo monthly monitoring as a precaution.

Current Investigations

Cytoxan® (Cyclophoshamide)

The use of Cytoxan is actively being studied for treatment of lung fibrosis. One recent study suggested that treating lung problems early on with this immunosuppressive drug might help prevent further damage and increase the chances of survival.

There is currently a two-year clinical trial underway that will try to measure the effectiveness of Cytoxan to control the progressive lung damage caused by scleroderma. Cytoxan works as an anti-inflammatory that also suppresses the immune system. It has been used for years in the treatment of leukemia and lymphoma. The drug has also shown promise treating arthritis and lupus.

The two-year trial will involve one hundred and sixty-three patients nationwide. All must have a moderate amount of lung damage. 50 percent will receive Cytoxan; the rest will receive a placebo. If the condition of a patient who is getting the placebo deteriorates during the study, they will be given the option of switching to cyclophoshamide. The drug has side effects and risks.[25]

Halofuginone

The Food and Drug Administration (FDA) has given orphan drug status for the development of Halofuginone in the treatment of scleroderma. Halofuginone is a specific inhibitor of collagen type I synthesis. A topical formulation is currently undergoing clinical trials in the UK. U.S. studies are still in the planning stages.

Halofuginone's consideration as a possible treatment for scleroderma had strange beginnings, even by scleroderma standards. It emerged when it was discovered that a chicken feed additive that contained halofuginone caused a chicken's skin to become fragile. Apparently, it prevented the chickens from synthesizing collagen. Aside from scleroderma, the drug is also being considered in treating cancer.

Uniprost

The FDA has granted a New Drug Application (NDA) for Uniprost, also known as Remodulin, a pulmonary hypertension drug. In a clinical trial involving about five hundred patients, the patient uses a beeper-size device that pumps medicine through the skin. Investigations are continuing.

Oral Collagen

At the time of publication, this NIH sponsored clinical trial was actively recruiting patients to find out if taking Type I Collagen by mouth will improve diffuse systemic sclerosis. It will involve 168 patients who will either receive type I collagen (made from cows) or a placebo, for twelve months.

Chapter 1

There has been new interest in an old drug with an infamous past. Thalidomide was responsible for one of the worst pharmaceutical disasters in history, when, in the 1950s and 60s, it was prescribed as an anti-nausea and sleep aid for pregnant women in Europe; it caused severe birth defects in about 10,000 babies.

Now, Thalidomide seems to be trying to overcome its past, and might be useful in a wide variety of diseases. Early results appear promising with some diseases, such as myeloma and certain types of ulcers. It has been a disappointment in others, like macular degeneration. For scleroderma, there are indications that it might be of some benefit. At this time, research is continuing.[26]

UK researchers are investigating the possible benefits of controlling the natural hormone serotonin in treating Raynaud's Phenomenon.[27] The investigation was initiated by the UK's Raynaud's and Scleroderma Association,[28] when it conducted an unofficial study that used ginko biloba, which naturally contains serotonin. Currently, investigators are following up with an official study that uses fluoxetine (Prozac®, normally prescribed for depression), which also contains certain properties that control the level of serotonin. Early results indicate that the frequency and severity of Raynaud's attacks are reduced.

Iloprost is currently being studied in Europe as a treatment for pulmonary hypertension. A French study of five patients showed some promise in the use of an inhaled form of the drug for patients awaiting lung and lung/heart transplants.

For information on other clinical studies, or, if you are interested in participating in a clinical trial, contact the NIH for current areas of investigation.[29]

The Business of Research

Scleroderma research is riddled with short-lived euphoric hopes. The story of Relaxin was especially discouraging. A July 4, 2000 New York Times headline hailed it as "A Weapon Found to Fight Scleroderma." By October 2000, it was just another false hope.[30]

The failure of Relaxin also showed how medical research is dependent upon the expectations of corporate profits. It was disappointing for patients to see the clinical trial fail, but the biggest problem faced by the manufacturer, Connetics Corporation, was the fury of its stockholders. The day that it announced that the "trial did not meet the primary outcome measurement for scleroderma," the company's stock became the stock market's loser-of-the-day, declining over 75 percent in value from the previous day's close.

The company also lost commitments of support from all of their international partners, from Japan to Europe. It was a classic example of the role that profits play in drug research programs.

Chapter 2

Finding The Right Doctor

Before scleroderma, you might have chosen a doctor based on bedside manner, on his or her willingness to write prescriptions for the drugs of your choice, or even because you were comfortable and on a first name basis with each other. The doctor-patient experience can make you feel vulnerable as soon as you enter an exam room so maybe your decisions were based only on what made you comfortable.

Although your comfort level with a doctor is very important, with scleroderma, comfort shouldn't be your only criteria. The doctor that was right for you before your diagnosis may not be the best one for you now.

Your role now requires a more collaborative relationship with a doctor that is receptive to your needs. This chapter is not only about finding the right doctor, but is also about how to be a better, more responsive patient. It is also an opportunity for you to decide the level of involvement you want in managing your disease. It's time to assess those needs and learn how to evaluate your current doctors, as well as future ones.

After the Diagnosis

In the beginning, getting a diagnosis can seem like the most difficult part of having scleroderma. It can drag on for months and even years. Not having a diagnosis can create unbearable stress. Unfortunately, due to the uncertainties of scleroderma, the stress doesn't necessarily go away after the diagnosis either.

In Karen's case, the disease progressed with unusual speed—she had only a few weeks before getting a diagnosis. The downside to a quick diagnosis is that it sometimes indicates a more rapid progression of the disease.

Sometimes the only advantage of getting a quick diagnosis is to validate that you are sick even though you may not look it to others. You are able to put a name on it, thereby knowing that what you are feeling is real and not just in your head. But contrary to instinctively feeling a sense of finality, it can be just the beginning of a difficult journey.

Karen initially had two issues that were important to her after her diagnosis. The first was to know that her rheumatologist was experienced in the disease. The second was to find out what the doctor's approach was to treatment and overall disease management.

A doctor who was filling in for her regular primary care physician referred her to a rheumatologist. From her initial visit, the rheumatologist seemed very concerned about her and showed a lot of sympathy. Usually, Karen liked sympathy from a doctor. But now, she knew she needed more than just sympathy. Karen asked a lot of questions, including the number of scleroderma patients the doctor was currently treating. She also wanted to know why all sorts of very strange and painful things were happening to her. Karen was not happy with the doctor's response. She felt that the answers were vague. From her perspective, the doctor either didn't know or was not being upfront—it had a very negative impact on her. She soon determined that this was not the doctor for her.

Aside from direct answers, what Karen really wanted to hear was any kind of assurance that her worst fears were not true. Of course, no doctor was going to be able to do that. After three months, she got a new rheumatologist, one that communicated very clearly and gave her confidence that he had the experience she wanted.

But as far as his approach to treatment was concerned, Karen was disappointed. He didn't suggest anything new that she wasn't already aware of. I think she was secretly hoping for some magic he was saving just for her. He was, though, open to most other treatments and medications that we brought to his attention. I don't think he really believed any of these would work, but maybe he figured there wasn't much risk to any of them either.

Where Do Doctors Come From?

Medical students are trained to help people, and a doctor has many ways to help. Some are best suited to working in a research environment, having little patient contact. Others are better in the traditional role of treating patients. Ideally, a scleroderma patient needs a doctor with a balance of both: one that has the curiosity of a researcher, and also a strong focus on the needs of the patient.

Many of the attributes that patients are looking for in doctors are put to the test in medical schools; patient skills don't seem to be necessary in becoming a doctor. Becoming de-sensitized to human need and emotion is not uncommon during this process. It's understandable and probably unavoidable. Working on cadavers certainly doesn't do much to develop patient skills, nor does the death they see during their residency. They sleep deprived, exhausted, and overwhelmed by the workload. As a result, many seem to end up focusing on the diagnosis and treatment rather than the patient.

As an example, in 2000, Karen had a medical crisis and was rushed to the hospital. Upon arrival at the ER, an intern that looked as though she had already been working twenty-four hours greeted us. For the next twenty hours that I saw her, she was always focused, but looked incredibly fatigued. It seemed that any human contact would have interfered. I had no complaints about her performance. But it was scary seeing someone in that position, being pushed to the edge of exhaustion. It's not likely that these kinds of grueling hours aid an intern's sensitivity to the needs of patients.

There are undoubtedly many medical students that survive residency with their focus still on the patient; however, such attentiveness just doesn't seem to be a requirement in becoming a doctor. The other side of the issue is when a doctor is too sensitive, or overly identifies with a patient (reminding them of a mother, wife, brother, etc.). It can impair their medical judgment. A happy medium is preferred.

How Patients Prevent Doctors From Doing Their Job

According to the American Society of Internal Medicine,[31] 70 percent of a correct diagnosis depends solely on what the patient tells the doctor. Giving doctors and other healthcare providers as much information as possible about your health, before and after being diagnosed with scleroderma, can provide faster, more accurate decisions about your health care needs.

In addition to the problem of doctors receiving accurate information, rambling patients who don't get to their point can hamper a doctor's effort. Some patients talk about things the doctor has no control over, and continuously repeat questions because they didn't get the answer they wanted the first time. Just as a patient needs a doctor that communicates clearly, the doctor needs the same from the patient.

Define Your Role

You can't ask yourself what you expect from your doctor until you know what you expect of yourself first.

Today, scleroderma has no cure. Finding a doctor that will put you back the way you were is probably not likely. But it doesn't, and shouldn't, stop most from trying. You need to understand how much information you can handle and understand the risks involved before you push the limits of treatment.

How active do you want to be in the decision making process with your doctor? It's up to each individual patient. Some (hopefully few) patients might say "you're the doctor, why ask me?" This book isn't going to be of much use to them. Others might constantly chase any kind of cure-in-a-bottle without understanding the risk. This book continuously encourages you to be as informed as possible and to consult your doctor before making any decisions that affects your health.

Most patients are somewhere in the middle of these two extremes. Defining yourself as a patient is an individualized process and has a lot to do with how informed you are and your temperament and personality. Whatever you decide, be comfortable with your decision.

When Defining Your Role, Consider the Following:
- Recognize the importance of a good doctor-patient relationship.
- Be as self-reliant as you can.
- Ask questions and communicate your needs.
- Recognize the impact of your life-style on your personal health.
- Do not depend solely on what the doctor can do for you.
- Take charge of your health in a way that fits with who you are.

Be a Good Patient
- Be honest.
- Open two-way communication.
- Mutually agreed upon goals.
- Let the doctor know what you expect of him.
- Let the doctor know what he can expect from you.

Considerations in Choosing a Doctor

Most likely, you already have a doctor. Maybe you're thinking about divorcing your current one and finding a new one. Use this section to see how your current or potential physician measures up. Your doctor needs to be your medical advisor and a partner that you can work with. Above all, you must have confidence in your doctor's overall ability. The doctor must be able to share your expectations, and must ultimately help your state of health.

Some Key Points
- Are you comfortable talking with your doctor?
- Does the doctor have a naturally curious nature?
- Are experimental and alternative treatments considered?
- Is there mutual agreement on the role you want him to play?
- What are your options in communicating?
  Is the doctor willing to take your phone calls to discuss specific issues that come up?
  Is the doctor willing to communicate through e-mail?
- What are the doctor's credentials? Medical school, hospital training, teaching staff, board certifications.
- Availability, the ease of making appointments.
- Does your insurance cover all the services and treatments?
- Is the doctor taking on new patients?

How to Find a New Doctor

A rheumatologist or dermatologist often is the one that manages a scleroderma patient's case, but the role of the primary care physician is also vital, especially in working with your specialist on the day-to-day issues. Sometimes the type of health insurance coverage you have will determine a doctor's role (discussed further in the next chapter). This section applies primarily to finding the specialist, but the same approach can be used to find a family practice physician as well.

In Karen's case, we depended upon her rheumatologist, initially, but, as the need for daily access to the medical system increased, the family practitioner became more involved. Karen was very lucky, because we already had a good relationship with our family doctor. A year and a half into Karen's disease, we asked him to be our point man, advisor, and conduit to the entire health care system. I doubt that he knew what he was getting into. He ended up going far beyond the call of duty in making himself accessible by phone and email, and most importantly, was willing to spend a massive amount of time dealing with the monstrous piles of paperwork required by managed care.

Compared to long-term patients, the newly diagnosed have a far more difficult time trying to anticipate what they'll need from a doctor. It takes experience to openly communicate and develop a good patient-doctor relationship. But before you decide what you want from a doctor, you have to weed through many other issues, like finding one that is local and accepts your health insurance plan (discussed more in Chapter 3).

There are many considerations in choosing a doctor, but the most important is their experience in treating scleroderma. Their level of experience with the disease not only is reflected in the treatments they recommend, but also will make it more likely that they can refer you to support groups. They should also be able to tell you what is happening with the latest in research. Their response to these questions will let you know their experience level with the disease.

Talking to other scleroderma patients can be a good way to learn about scleroderma specialists. The best ways are either through a local support group[32] or the Internet (online support is discussed later in Chapter 5). What you have to consider, though, is that another patient's criteria for getting a doctor may not be the same as yours. Also, on the Internet, you don't have the advantage of seeing the people first-hand, or really knowing anything more than what they want you to know.

Sometimes, newly diagnosed patients, who stand to gain the most by contacting other patients, are the most reluctant to do so. It might be that they are still very much in denial and unable to deal with the disease. Karen didn't want to go to our local support group meeting, at first because she was afraid to see the faces that she thought would represent her future. Later, because of the speed and severity of her case, she didn't want to make anyone feel uncomfortable in thinking that she represented their future. By the time she did go, a year and a half after diagnosis, we had already gone through the process of finding doctors on our own (and as usual, it was the hard way).

If your local resources don't get you anywhere, contact a scleroderma organization.[32] [33] They will not guarantee the right doctor for you, but they are usually able to refer you to experienced scleroderma doctors in your area. Becoming a member or making a donation to one of these organizations will also get you on their newsletter mailing list and will help keep you abreast of recent developments. Their websites and newsletters might also list or profile scleroderma specialists or medical advisory board members who might be geographically close to you. If none of them are near you, it's possible that one of these doctors might be able to recommend a specialist in your area. You can even search for specialists that have been published.[34]

These are creative ways of seeking the right doctor. For most of us, regardless of the type of health insurance you have, a more practical way is to check out a doctor directory at the American College of Rheumatology,[35] American Medical Association,[36] or other organizations listed in the next section. You will be able to look for doctors in the specialty you want, by city or zip code, insurance plan, or hospital.

Once you've selected three or four doctors, it's time to take a closer look. Always double-check any information from the Internet, even if it is from a respected organization. There is little to protect you from misinformation except your own good judgment.

WHERE TO CHECK CREDENTIALS

American Medical Association (AMA)
    The AMA website allows you to check training, certificates and a doctor's biographical information. From its homepage, go to patients, then doctor finder. You can look for a doctor's specialty, hospital, and affiliation.

American Board Of Medical Specialty[37]
    The American Board of Medical Specialties can tell you if the doctor is board certified. "Certified" means that the doctor has completed a training program in a specialty and has passed an exam (board) to assess his or her knowledge, skills, and experience to provide quality patient care in that specialty. Primary care doctors also may be certified as specialists. While board certification is a good measure of a doctor's knowledge, it is possible to receive quality care from doctors who are not board certified.

Chapter 2

Administrators in Medicine[38]

This website is run by AIM, the Administrators in Medicine Association of State Medical Board Executive Directors. It will refer you to your home state medical board, and provides the doctor's education, date graduated, if their license is current, and state license number. Only about half of the states participate in this organization, but it's growing. State medical boards currently offer the best opportunity to see any enforcement that has been taken against a doctor. If your state is not listed, get the phone number of your state medical board from a local phone book and contact it directly.

American College of Rheumatology[39]

This is a very useful site because it not only lists rheumatologists geographically, but also lists practicing physicians, research scientists, nurses, physical and occupational therapists, psychologists, and social workers that are connected to rheumatology. The site also lists each person's discipline, such as patient care, research, teaching, or government. Not only helpful for patients in the U.S, it lists doctors worldwide. International rheumatology links are also available at the site.

Public Citizen's Health Research Group[40]

Want to know if a doctor has ever been disciplined? It's not easy information to get. It is said that the government's National Practitioner Data Bank (NPDB) has more than a quarter of a million adverse records on nearly 150,000 health care practitioners, mostly physicians. Unfortunately, it is not available to the public. Public Citizen's has comprised its own list, which it sells for $20. One of its complaints (one of many—see their website), in addition to not allowing public access to the database, is that doctors who have been disciplined for narcotics-related offenses can voluntarily give up their federal narcotics license so they won't be included in government reports.

They say that doctors "usually" give up their licenses only when revocation is imminent.

First Visit

After you have narrowed your list of doctors, the next step is to schedule a visit with the doctor of your choice. During that first visit you will learn a lot about the doctor's style of communication and how it fits with yours. When communicating with the doctor, each of your respective personal styles will tend to indicate if there is an ability to work together.

At your meeting, make sure the doctor already has your medical records, or carry them in with you. You will need to say why you are looking for a new doctor, how you ended up seeing him, and what doctor qualities are important to you. The doctor needs to know your goals for both the short and long term, and the level of involvement you want in managing your disease. You can open with this, or listen to what he has to say first; either way, the doctor needs to know your agenda early on.

Be prepared with the following (not only on the first visit, but with every doctor appointment):

- If you need physical or emotional assistance, bring a friend or family member.
- A written list of points you want to cover.
- Be honest.
- Be prepared to provide an accurate personal and family medical history. (Chapter 3, PMO)
- Always have a current list of medication, including any dietary supplements or alternative therapies. (Chapter 3, PMO)
- Take notes that will become a part of your personal records (Chapter 3, PMO).
- Make sure you understand the doctor's medical assessment, and options.

- Find out if the options discussed are covered by your insurance.
- Know the risks associated with specific treatments that you are interested in.
- Inform the doctor if you feel unable to follow any suggested treatments or medications.
- Do not leave without fully understanding what the doctor has said.

Trust your own reactions when deciding whether this doctor is the right one for you. You also may want to give the relationship some time to develop. It takes more than one visit for you and your doctor to get to know each other.

Wrap up of First Appointment

How did the doctor do?
1. Were you given a chance to ask questions? Yes-No
2. Did the doctor really listen to your questions? Yes-No
3. Were answers given in terms you understood? Yes-No
4. Were you shown respect? Yes-No
5. Were you asked pertinent questions? Yes-No
6. Did the doctor make you feel comfortable? Yes-No
7. Did the doctor address all your questions? Yes-No
8. Were you asked if you had treatment preferences? Yes-No
9. Did the doctor spend enough time with you? Yes-No

If you think this is the doctor for you, make sure to assess the office staff as well.

Chapter 3

Managing Your Care

In retrospect, twenty-five years ago seemed like a happier time for patients, doctors, hospitals, and insurance companies. Back then, patients simply complained to doctors about their high medical bills, doctors would wonder what the problem was because it was covered by insurance; insurance companies would generally pay the claims without question; and patients would complain that the insurance companies kept raising their premiums.

Since then, there has been a continuing power struggle between these groups. Each has tried to shove the cost of health onto the others. During the 1980s, Medicare clamped down; in the 1990s, managed care put the pressure on doctors and hospitals—and the patient got caught in the middle.

Now, managed care companies are running out of ideas to reduce their costs. Whatever is tried, the patient seems to get squeezed more and more. For scleroderma patients, health insurance issues are occupying time that would be better spent on the personal side of improving their health, not contending with the medical bureaucracy.

Unfortunately, there's no escaping these issues. They not only affect the cost of coverage, but also the potential quality of the patient-doctor relationship.

Personal Medical Organizers

There is no tool that can help you become a better self-directed patient than a Personal Medical Organizer (PMO). It can be the cornerstone in managing your disease.

A PMO is your own medical record. It includes information your doctor would normally have, plus allows for your own input. It keeps you focused and organized, saves time, and helps you do a better job in communicating your needs to your doctor (example on page 44).

Some scleroderma patients have always kept their own medical records. It's not a new concept, and it comes more naturally to some than others. It can make an important difference in managing any disease. A PMO is especially important for scleroderma patients because it can assist the doctor by providing better information that can help zero-in on the patient's specific needs. Scleroderma can be erratic, with alternating cycles of flare-ups and low activity. A PMO gives you a better chance to understand what is happening and stay on top of it.

Each scleroderma patient is different. Each decides the level of involvement they want in managing their disease. Each has certain areas that are more important to be involved in than others. These differences can be reflected in how you set up your own PMO. You should do it in a way that makes the most sense to you.

In Karen's case, there were dozens of problems that perhaps could have been controlled better but which simply got out of hand. There always seemed to be too many fires to contain at once, and sometimes we couldn't tell the potentially big problems from the small ones. A PMO allows you to see the bigger picture and is easier to convey the situation to your doctor.

As an example, seven months after her diagnosis, Karen had an ulcer on the middle knuckle of her middle finger. It not only wouldn't heel, but gradually got bigger. We came close to healing it a couple of times, then we lost our focus to other problems. She ended up having the knuckle surgically removed, and the bone fused. During surgery, she was given too much fluid. Her lungs filled up and she ended up in congestive heart failure. They used heavy doses of diuretics to remove the fluid from the lungs and around the heart. Although her kidney function started declining months before, the diuretics (in my opinion) put more stress on her kidneys, causing them to fail (at least prematurely). Within a few weeks she was on kidney dialysis. Kidney dialysis was one of the hardest things for her to endure. I have often wondered what might have happened if we had been able to heal that ulcer in the first place.

There can be several parts to your PMO. Each of these parts are explained below. Customize it to suit your condition and needs, so it helps support you in how you want to manage your disease.

The PMO can be handwritten in a 3-ringed binder that is divided into the sections you want, or it can be pre-printed forms that you buy.[41] [42] It can even be organized and saved in simple "Word" type document folders on your PC just the way it is organized below. Specialized PMO software programs are also available for your computer[43] and Palm Pilots (PDA), along with free trials and shareware.[44] Whatever you decide, be comfortable with your choice.

The following is an outline of the structure of a PMO. An example of what a PMO actually looks like can be seen at the Scleroderma Press website.[45]

Part I— Medical History
Personal and medical information, family history.

Part II— Tests & Lab Reports
Blood, imaging, lung function, GI, baseline tests.

Part III— Insurance Information.
Copy of policy, contact information.

Part IV— Copy of Doctor & Hospital Records.
Some doctors prefer to withhold medical records because they don't think patients will understand or interpret them accurately. As part of picking the right doctor, he should already understand your motivations and priorities. (See patient rights)

Part V— Calendar of Appointments

Part VI— Advance Directive
See information at the end of this chapter.

Part VII— Medical Diary
The Medical Diary is your own record of any event that you feel necessary to record. Your diary can help you and your doctor do a better job of identifying problems.

Part VIII— Doctor Appointment Checklist
The checklist has two purposes. First, the patient records all concerns and questions before an appointment (not a bad idea to start this list several days before an appointment). Secondly, the patient takes notes on the doctor's responses to each point and indicates how satisfactory the response was. You should have an appointment checklist for every healthcare provider appointment (including alternative care providers).

Part IX— Phone and E-mail Records
Note all communication with healthcare providers.

Part X— Scleroderma Research

What do you do with news stories about scleroderma or when you hear something interesting about the disease from someone else? Organize it. You can save it in a scrapbook, or scan it into your computer; either way manages your information so you can use it when you need it.

Part XI— Medication Management

Medications mean all prescription drugs and over-the-counter products, as well as alternative treatments, such as vitamins and herbs. Your doctor should know everything you're taking (Chapter 4).

Prescription Costs

Regardless of whether you have good insurance, or bad insurance, it's better than no insurance. For those patients that are unable to afford either the drugs or the cost of insurance, there are ways you can reduce your out-of-pocket expense. A good place to start is by checking out the Pharmaceutical Research and Manufacturers of America.[46] They have a program in which you can get certain prescriptions at a reduced cost, or, even at no cost. Each member drug company has its own program and criteria. After approval, medications are usually sent directly to your doctor for pickup.

Another option is to buy your drugs outside the United States. The rest of the world knows that Americans pay more than anybody else for drugs, and that's why many foreign drug companies try to sell us back the drugs that were originally manufactured in the U.S. Canada has been a favorite for filling American prescriptions for those with no insurance, and it is said that the typical savings can range from 30 percent to 70 percent. Canadian Internet sites that offer mail order service are also gaining popularity. If you choose this route, keep your doctor informed.

Many doctors are often unaware of the costs of medications or insurance issues. Let your doctor know what is covered and what isn't. Often times the patient gets caught in the middle between a doctor that is prescribing medication based on his medical judgment and demands from managed care that pressure the doctor to choose, based on cost.

It is not always clear what medication is best for you. Most drugs have one or more alternatives that produce similar results, but work differently. The same drug tends to work a little bit differently in each patient, with varying degrees of therapeutic value and side effects. For Karen's GI involvement, she was prescribed Prilosec, which was considered best in its class, and was fully covered by our insurance. The only problem was it really didn't work very well for her. For a brief time, she found that Protonix, a similar drug, which cost 30 percent less at the time, worked better. So work with your doctor to constantly fine-tune what is best, both in terms of cost and effectiveness.

MEDICAL INSURANCE OVERVIEW

Understanding insurance issues can be like trying to learn a foreign language. Unfortunately, you can't properly manage your care without having a basic understanding of your insurance coverage and what it takes to make it work. The good news is that you don't have to be an expert. The following information will help you learn what you need to know.[47]

Considering what special features you need in a health insurance policy is a moot point for those that are struck and unable to change their existing coverage. Perhaps this section will provide options that weren't previously considered.

For others who are in a position to change their health insurance policy, it is important to understand the difference between one insurance policy and another in being able to meet any special needs you may have.

Because of scleroderma's erratic nature, it's not always easy to determine what you might need in addition to customary benefits. Common areas that do need consideration, though, are durable medical equipment, coverage for "alternative treatments" and special procedures, knowing what drugs are not covered, grievance procedures, and, most importantly, the ability to see doctors that are experienced with scleroderma.

Second Opinions

Any serious diagnosis or procedure is reason enough to have the ability to get a second opinion. It informs you and can make you feel more secure with your decisions—it's peace of mind.

Asking for a second opinion can be uncomfortable for some, but it's best to stay focused on your care, and not the doctor's feelings. Besides, second opinions are a routinely accepted practice by most doctors. When seeking a second opinion, be honest with your doctor about your reasons. The doctor will have to forward your records so don't avoid it.

If your doctor does take offense or tries to discourage you, this doctor may not be for you. Also, you need an independent and balanced view; don't go to the doctor next door (if you can avoid it) and try and get someone out of your doctor's network. Faced with the same facts, competent doctors often disagree. If you get an opinion that conflicts sharply with the first, have the two doctors confer with each other so they can thoroughly explain their differences to you.

The formality of getting a second opinion varies from Health Maintenance Organizations (HMO) to Preferred Provider Organizations (PPO), and from state to state. In general, a PPO allows you a variety of choices but will usually have an additional co-pay. In an HMO, you need your PCP to authorize a second opinion; it will probably be within their network of doctors and maybe even in the same building. This is one way an HMO can limit your choice. If a PCP doesn't want to give you a referral, you will probably have to file a grievance in accordance with the terms of your policy.

Insurance Benefits

Most of us depend upon the insurance marketing brochure to tell us what is covered, and, usually, that is enough. But you have the right to see the complete medical insurance contract, before you buy, and after. But each state may vary in the procedure necessary to get your own copy. If your health insurance is through your employer, they will most likely have a copy in their head office. These policies are also on file in your local state office, usually at the Department of Insurance or Department of Corporations. If there is any difficulty in obtaining a copy, contact your local state legislator.

Certain procedures, like stem cell transplants, could be a battle to get covered by any insurance policy. Yet there are others, even if unproven, that might be covered. At the urging of one friend, and the help from another, Karen underwent plasmaphoresis, an unproven therapy for scleroderma that some say can stop the progression of the disease. In this particular case, Karen's policy covered the same list of treatments that are approved by Medicare, and surprisingly, plasmaphoresis was on Medicare's list. In any case, it is necessary to be aware of what treatments are covered. If you are locked into a health policy and are unable to change, at least know what your coverage does offer.

Rating Health of Insurance Companies

Judging the quality of a health plan is not a science. Today's plans include a variety of options; you need to understand what you want versus its cost in order to choose what's right for you.

A good place to look for information that evaluates managed care, hospital statistics by medical specialty, or how your HMO ranks, is the U.S. News and World Report Guide[48] and the National Opinion Research Center.[49]

Checking out an insurance plan is not difficult, but there is no universal standard for comparisons. All of the organizations listed below rate the quality of health insurance companies, and if you browse around each of the sites, you will find a lot of other useful information. Some offer accreditations; others use their own scorecard to measure quality.

The four major organizations that track and compare health insurance are as follows: the National Committee for Quality Assurance;[50] the Accreditation Association for Ambulatory Health Care;[51] the Joint Commission on Accreditation of Healthcare Organizations;[52] and the American Accreditation Health Care Commission.[53]

After you have checked out a plan's quality care rating, it's just as important to rate its financial health. Many HMOs, PPOs and other types of insurers are having significant financial problems, and a number of them are going out of business. Generally, patients and their families are protected under state laws against financial responsibility for medical bills in the event a health plan becomes insolvent. However, there are some instances where a patient can be stuck with financial obligations, so it is important to investigate the plan you choose. You can get financial ratings from the following companies: Standard and Poor's,[54] A.M. Best,[55] Moody's Investors Service,[56] and Weiss Ratings.[57]

Changing Medical Insurance After Being Diagnosed

Maybe you would like to change your health insurance coverage. Unfortunately, you are limited once you've been diagnosed and might even have lost the ability to change your insurance plan altogether. But there are some general exceptions to this. In addition, there may be specific exceptions that apply only in your home state.

As a general rule, the best chance of changing your insurance after diagnosis is if you already have health insurance through your employer. The employer plan may allow you to change from an HMO to a PPO, or there might be an open enrollment period for a new plan offering.

Another way to change insurance is while changing jobs. You have the same choices in accepting employee health plan options as anyone else; however, you may have to disclose your diagnosis as a pre-existing condition and may have a waiting period until it becomes active. Make sure you know what applies to your situation.

A note of caution . . .

If you are eligible for Medicare, sometimes an employer or healthcare provider will advise you to drop your existing health insurance and switch to Medicare. Be careful and get good advice from someone who knows the rules. It's possible that it is not in *your* best interest but in your employer's for you to change. If after looking into it, you conclude that it is a good move for you, be aware that you will be prematurely using certain lifetime Medicare benefits that have a cap. Also, unless you have a supplemental policy, Medicare does not cover prescriptions.

Having an individual health insurance plan is another matter. Unfortunately, there is no general formula for being able to change insurance. Do some research on the subject, and if necessary, you can call your state legislator for assistance.

BASIC TYPES OF HEALTH INSURANCE

The traditional medical, Fee-For-Service plan profile

- Having complete freedom to choose doctors and hospitals is the most important, even if it costs more.

- Being able to choose any doctor or hospital in the country.

- Not minding to fill out forms or keeping receipts and sending them in for reimbursement.

- Willing to pay for the cost of routine and preventive care, such as checkups and shots.

- More likely to get an office appointment when you want one.

- Deciding what specialist you want to see and when.

- Don't want to have to see a primary care doctor each time before a specialist is seen.

If this fits you, then you want the traditional kind of health care policy. Insurance companies pay fees for the services provided to the insured people covered by their policies. This type of health insurance offers the greatest choice of doctors and hospitals. You can choose any doctor you wish and change doctors at any time. You can go to any hospital in any part of the country. You will usually pay a certain percentage of your bill as either a deductible or as a co-payment.

In a typical plan, the deductible might be $250 for each person in your family, with a family deductible of $500 when at least two people in the family have reached the individual deductible. Not all health expenses you have count toward your deductible.

To receive payment for claims, you have to fill out forms and send them to your insurer. You are responsible for keeping track of receipts for all medical costs, including drugs.

Chapter 3

Health Maintenance Organization Profile (HMO)

- Keeping down cost is most important, even if it means limiting some choices.

- Generally restricted to medical care in your own geographic area.

- Requires the least amount of paper work.

- Provides routine and preventive care.

- Okay to have to wait for services to be scheduled.

- Not a problem to see the primary care doctor first to be referred to specialists.

HMOs are the ultimate example of managed care. As an HMO member, you pay a monthly premium in exchange for doctor visits, hospital stays, emergency care, surgery, lab tests, x-rays, and therapy. There may also be a small co-payment for each office visit, prescription or ER visit. Your total medical costs will likely be lower and more predictable in an HMO than with the traditional fee-for-service insurance.

In almost all HMOs, you are either assigned, or you choose one doctor to serve as your PCP. This doctor monitors your health and provides most of your medical care, referring you to specialists and other health care professionals as needed. You usually cannot see a specialist without a referral from your PCP, who is expected to manage most of the care you receive.

Some people think that managed care should really be called managed cost. The theory behind an HMO is that the doctor receives a fixed amount of money per month, regardless of the number of office visits, so it is in the doctor's interest to make sure you get basic health care for problems before they become serious. The fixed fee is called "capitation." A typical capitation fee is $9 per month per patient. With this kind of financial structure, it's easy to understand why many HMO doctor groups have gone out of business.

To make sure HMOs don't cut costs at the expense of the patient's health, federal and state governments have tried to regulate certain procedures. The courts, on the other hand, have tended to affirm an HMO's right to "ration" care, indicating that there are limits of care an HMO is obligated to provide a patient. This rationing of care is the reality of HMO policies, even though there is an effort to make sure that the quality of care is not sacrificed too much.

New and proposed state laws are addressing this issue. A recent news article[58] profiled the effort of forty-one states that mandate some sort of outside review for handling HMO complaints. California is the largest HMO market, and is at the forefront of this trend. The state created the Department of Managed Health Care in 2000, with many feeling that it offers the best glimpse of how patient rights will rollout in the rest of the country.

Most of these state laws were designed to protect the patient, especially in life-threatening situations. But most state review processes allow an insurance company to use the advantage of their legal resources to refute claims made by the patient. It often can turn into a "you said/they said" contest. The primary disadvantage to the patient is that the insurance company has the "official" medical records, complete with notes. The patient has nothing but memory to depend upon (unless they have a PMO to support their claims). A PMO helps level the playing field during times of dispute.

Karen was covered by an HMO policy. It took many years for her to be convinced that we should switch from a fee-for-service plan. Just a year before she got sick, we signed on to an HMO that had the UCLA Medical Center network as a provider. Its high rating and the fact that it was a teaching hospital was what finally convinced her.

In the end, our experience with an HMO was good. We had access to scleroderma specialists, and, although there was much more red tape for the doctor, I never got the impression that her HMO insurance affected the overall care and treatment she received. As pointed out in the last chapter, I believe that the ultimate reason for Karen's good care had more to do with the dedication and excellent relationship with her doctors and other healthcare professionals than the type of insurance she had.

Preferred Provider Organization (PPO)

Preferred Provider Organizations are somewhere between an HMO and a traditional fee-for-service plan. The PPO is the least restrictive of the managed care plans. PPO doctors are not capitated, but there is less emphasis on preventative care. The position of the primary care physician is similar to their status in an HMO, but there is also a wider network of doctors to choose from. But one of the main advantages of a PPO is that you can use a doctor or specialist outside of the network. If you utilize this feature, the PPO will only pay a portion of the costs, but at least you have the choice.

Alternative Treatment

Traditionally, fee-for-service, PPOs or HMOs have not covered most alternative treatments. That is changing. Almost all of the major health insurance companies either have, or are planning to add, at least some alternative care.

Blue Cross of California is in the process of getting state approval for its "ultra premier" plan. It will allow twenty-four visits a year to an acupuncturist, $300 worth of massage treatment, $300 toward a health club membership and $500 for any herbal medicines. The policy will cost considerably more than the typical policy.

Aetna has a "natural alternatives" program, offering a wide range of services, including massage and nutritional counseling. Aetna says the alternative provider information on its website gets more "hits" than any other part of the site, including its doctor and hospital lists.

Medicare

Medicare is the federal health insurance program for Americans age sixty-five and older and can also apply to scleroderma patients who are disabled. Today, nearly 38 million people receive Medicare assistance.

Medicare has two parts: hospital insurance, known as Part A, and supplementary medical insurance, known as Part B, which provides payments for doctors and related services and supplies ordered by the doctor. If you are eligible for Medicare, Part A has no premium, Part B does. Medicare has very limited benefits for long-term care services and no benefits for prescription drugs. Medicare operates on a fee-for-service basis, and in some areas, through HMOs.[59] [60]

Medigap Insurance

Over 25 percent of the people who are covered by Medicare buy private insurance called "Medigap" policies, to pay the medical bills that Medicare doesn't cover. Some Medigap policies cover Medicare's deductibles; most pay the coinsurance amount. Some also pay for health services not covered by Medicare. There are ten standard plans from which you can choose, most of them available in every state.

Even with this insurance, there are still many "gaps" in health coverage. According to a recent report from the General Accounting Office,[61] only 8 percent of those buying standardized policies bought drug coverage (few carriers even offer plans with drug benefits).

Medicaid

Medicaid is a federal program that is operated by the states, and each state decides who is eligible and the scope of the health services offered. Medicaid provides health care coverage for certain low-income people who cannot afford regular health insurance. Medicaid is intended for people who have few assets, excluding their home, and often applies to people who have had to liquidate assets resulting from medical bills from a chronic or catastrophic illness. You can get an overview of this program from the federal website[62] or by contacting your home state office.

Medical Savings Accounts (Self-employed) [63]

The Medical Savings Account (MSA) is geared for the self-employed. It is based on a low premium and a high-deductible.

An MSA has two parts: catastrophic insurance coverage that kicks in after the deductible has been paid, and a savings account that can be tapped to pay the deductible. The attraction of this plan is a much lower health insurance premium, and a deductible that is paid out before it is taxed. Deductibles can range from $1,600 to $2,400 for an individual.

MSA's have some interesting features, including some cases where you can use it to cover expenses not covered by your health insurance, such as alternative treatments and even dental visits.

At the time this book was published, it was not certain if Congress would continue this program. There is currently a new proposed law to extend and expand this program. Anyone that has an existing MSA by the end of 2002 would be allowed to continue.

Health Care Spending Accounts (Employees)

As employers reduce the coverage and increase the deductibles of their employee health plans, Health Care Spending Accounts are becoming more popular. Eighty-five percent of the nation's large employers offer these plans. There is some similarity to the MSA in that it allows employees to set aside part of their pretax wages to pay their share of deductibles, co-payments, and sometimes non-covered treatments. Money is taken out before paycheck taxes. For scleroderma patients, it can also help reduce the cost of seeing specialists that are not covered through their basic insurance policy.

What Happens When You Can't Work Anymore?

One out of every seven workers will suffer a five-year or longer period of disability before age sixty-five, yet 65 percent of full-time workers in the private sector have no long-term disability income insurance, according to a 1998 Bureau of Labor Statistics report. Each year, more than 380,000 working-age Americans find themselves unable to work because of a long-term disability.

Soon after Karen was diagnosed with scleroderma in 1998, it became apparent she was not going to be able to continue working. For most of her life, she had paid little into the Social Security system because she was either doing volunteer charity fundraising or working in a family business. Fortunately, she had enough social security credits to qualify for Social Security Disability.

Shrinking income and rapidly increasing medical costs during a medical crisis is the last thing you need. It was a daunting task to determine our options, and difficult to find out what was available through state and federal programs.

Unfortunately, as far as insurance coverage is concerned, more of us are better prepared for death than for a chronic disability. Seventy-six percent of households own life insurance. But according to the American Council of Life Insurers,[64] people between the ages of thirty-five and sixty-five are much more likely to suffer a serious disability than to die. Further evidence of this is revealed in a U.S. Department of Housing and Urban Development report that states that 2 percent of all home foreclosures are due to deaths, while 46 percent are a result of disability.[65]

That leaves many of us to depend upon the "tattered safety net" provided by various government programs. The following outlines the concept of assistance available for the disabled through government and private insurance.

GOVERNMENT DISABILITY

State Programs

If you are unable to work as a result of scleroderma, your home state is where you first make a claim. As is the case with many issues, each state has its own requirements and standards. Contact your state disability office, or your local state legislator.

Federal Programs

Depending upon where you live, your state disability will probably run from six to eighteen months. Federal disability, under the Social Security Administration, requires a one year wait to come into play, but it is suggested that the application process start before then. Federal benefits can be difficult to get, especially for scleroderma patients that look fine on the outside, but are very sick inside. The government can be tough in recognizing a disability,[66] but, when they do, it can be for life.

Under this program, you can receive roughly what you would get at sixty-five on Social Security. A disability is defined as having lasted or expected to last at least one year, and prevents you from doing any substantial gainful work. If you have private disability insurance, you can simultaneously collect government and private policy benefits. After twenty-four months of disability you become eligible for Medicare (three months if on kidney dialysis).[67]

Supplemental Security Income (SSI)

Five million Americans receive SSI. It is operated jointly by the federal and state governments and is administered by the Social Security Administration. It is designed to guarantee a minimum income to the financially strapped and can include disabled scleroderma patients—if they have not worked enough to qualify for social security benefits. Monthly payments average $754 for an individual and $1,255 for a disabled worker that has a spouse and one child. If you qualify for SSI, you will probably qualify for Medicaid, food stamps, rehabilitation, and some home care services as well.[68]

GOVERNMENT PROTECTION OF BENEFITS

ERISA

If you are entitled to disability, health, life insurance, pension, severance, or almost any other type of benefit from your employer or union membership, a federal statute entitled the Employee Retirement Income Security Act of 1974 (ERISA), governs your rights to those benefits.

If you become disabled as a result of scleroderma and are unable to work, check out your rights under the rules of the benefits' plan. Any questions should first be directed to your employer's benefits manager. Any disputes should go to The Department's Pension and Welfare Benefits Administration (PWBA),[69] together with the Internal Revenue Service (IRS).[70]

COBRA

The Consolidated Omnibus Budget Reconciliation Act of 1986 (COBRA)[71] provides for a continuation of health insurance coverage to employees who were covered by group plans of twenty or more employees. These employers must offer participants and beneficiaries the option to continue group health coverage in the case of certain events (such as disability, terminating from a job or a change in family status) for eighteen to thirty-six months depending on the qualifying event.

The former employee may be required to pay the group rate premium plus a surcharge of up to two percent to cover administrative costs. Unfortunately, if unemployed, the premium can sometimes be too expensive.

HIPAA

HIPAA is the acronym for the Health Insurance Portability and Accountability Act of 1996. The Center for Medicare and Medicaid Services is responsible for implementing the many unrelated provisions of HIPAA, therefore HIPAA may mean different things to different people. As it applies to scleroderma patients, pre-existing medical conditions cannot exclude applicants from being hired and obtaining medical insurance. There can be, though, up to a six-month waiting period for benefits to kick-in.[72]

Long-Term Care Insurance

A long-term care insurance policy is primarily designed to cover the costs of nursing home care. Long-term care is usually not covered by other health insurance except in a very limited way. Medicare covers very few long-term care expenses. There are many types of long-term plans, and they vary in costs and services covered, with each having their own limits. These policies are written according to the regulations of each state.

Home Health Care Services

If you do need home healthcare services, make sure to check their accreditation.[73 74 75 76] An agency's credential for federal or state licensing and Medicare certification can be checked through the Joint Commission On Accreditation of Health Care Organizations.[77]

Let Your Will Be Known

Advance directives are best done well before an emergency. The purpose of an advance directive is to let the health care provider know the kind of medical care you want or don't want, should you become incapacitated. It can also relieve your family and friends of the responsibility for making decisions regarding life-prolonging actions.

In Karen's case, within six months of diagnosis, half a dozen doctors, and a cadre of social workers and home health service people were seeing her. Almost all of them started to talk about the need for an advance directive. I was suspicious and felt it was some sort of signal that they were giving up on her. I feared their concern was based more on economics than on quality of life issues.

Karen's own wishes were not unusual. She had stated things like, no heroic measures, do not resuscitate, no life support. But I was opposed to putting it in writing. I was afraid it might affect the decisions of doctors if there was a medical crisis when she was in the hospital with no family around. I don't know if that should have been a real fear or if I was just a little paranoid. We ended up having an advance directive that stated her wishes but left the ultimate decisions up to me.

There are two types of advance directives: A living will, which states your written wishes about what medical treatment you would not want if you be unable to communicate, and a medical power of attorney, a document that lets you appoint someone you trust to make decisions about your medical care if you cannot make decisions for yourself.

Your right to accept or refuse treatment is protected by constitutional common law, and by the federal Patient Self-Determination Act (PSDA),[78] which requires all health care facilities that receive Medicare or Medicaid funds to inform patients about their rights to refuse medical treatment or to sign an advance directive. Still, each state regulates the use of advance directives differently, and some physicians and hospitals are resistant to follow them.

For information and counseling on advance directives and state-specific forms that comply with local laws, contact the Partnership For Caring, Inc., a national non-profit organization.[79] If you need additional help in preparing an advance directive, or if you would like more information, you may want to contact a lawyer, a nearby hospital, or your state attorney general's office.

Advance directives are not required and may be canceled at any time. You do not have to prepare an advance directive if you do not want one but if you do choose to have one, the originals of living wills and advance directives should be signed and dated in accordance with state law, and copies should be given to your doctor and hospital; be sure to retain the original in your PMO. Some people even carry a small card in their wallet stating that they have an advance directive, where it is located, and who your agent or proxy is, if you have named one.

In Karen's case, the issue of advance directives was put to the test in 2000. While wrapping up a typical evening of watching television, her head started to hurt so badly she started to cry uncontrollably in pain. After forty-five minutes, she finally quieted down, seeming to sleep, but I could hear a strange noise coming from her chest. She picked her head up at one point, looked up to the ceiling as though she was seeing something of wonderment, and then closed her eyes again. Ten minutes later her body shuttered and convulsed repeatedly for three or four minutes.

The ambulance was quick. In the ER, the first thing they asked was if she had an advance directive. I said, without producing any paper, that she left the decisions about her care to me. They wanted to know her wishes about being on a ventilator (life support). Rather than answering the question, I asked what would happen if she wasn't hooked up to one; they said she would probably die within a few hours. I asked what was wrong with her; they said they didn't know. I asked how long she would be on the ventilator; they said they didn't know. I asked if it was possible that it would be only a day or two; they said yes. I asked if it was possible that she might never been taken off the ventilator; they said yes.

Literally following her wishes, I should have just stayed at her side and watched her die. I knew she didn't want to be on any form of life support, and I agreed, but that was meant to avoid being kept artificially alive in the long-term. We (maybe just me) weren't prepared at that time to make life and death decisions that weren't clear-cut. What if it was only a day, or a week, or even a month? I wasn't capable of letting her die if the ventilator was necessary for just a few weeks.

I gave the okay to put her on the ventilator. As it turned out, she had had a seizure. Ten days later, she came off the ventilator.

What did Karen think about all this when she finally opened her eyes? She was happy that everyone gathered around her was overjoyed to see her. Everybody felt it was a victory; but for Karen, she soon realized that nothing had changed; she still had scleroderma, but was now much weaker than before.

Patient Rights

New patient privacy regulations went into effect in April 2001 as part of HIPAA[80] regulations. It will require that health insurers and care providers obtain a patient's consent before using or revealing medical records for purposes of treatment, billing or other healthcare operations. Healthcare providers covered by these rules include doctors, dentists, hospitals, clinics, nurses, and pharmacists.

Before the adoption of these rules, patients in most states had no legal right to their own medical records. The new regulations now give everyone the right to see, copy and correct their health records.

The rules are effective now, but companies have a two-year grace period to bring their policies in line with the new rules. In most cases, the new rules will not be enforced until April 2003.

Chapter 4

Alternative

vs.

Mainstream Care

Before scleroderma, Karen was a mainstream kind of patient. Choosing medical care was a very simple process: she just put herself in the hands of the best doctor she could find, and did what she was told.

When she was diagnosed with scleroderma, she followed doctors orders and took all the usual drugs, including penicillamine, prednisone, methotrexate, cytoxan, and so on. They didn't help. She then tried medical therapies that were on the edge of mainstream medicine, like minocin, PUVA, and even plasmaphoresis.[81] When those didn't work either, she considered a stem cell transplant and the Relaxin clinical trials, but kidney failure prevented her from being a candidate for either. Each of these treatments seemed to offer hope for some, but not her.

During this time, her opinion of alternative medicine (treatments not usually recommended by doctors) began to change. She didn't really know much about it, but her traditionally negative views on the subject became more neutral, no longer looking upon it as some sort of New Age Voodoo. She didn't know if any alternative treatment could help, and she wasn't ready to strap on magnets just yet, but she *did* know that mainstream medicine wasn't working.

Her friends and family would have done anything to help—but weren't sure what to do. Surprisingly, many sent books, articles and emails (lots of them) on alternative treatments. She received a total of twenty-eight books, almost all dealing with alternative therapies. The subjects ranged from macrobiotics to the joys of juicing, Edgar Cayce's detailed accounts of how he cured several scleroderma patients, and several on herbal remedies. A faith healer and psychic were even sent to the house.

Before we get any further into exploring alternative therapies, please keep in mind that there are strong arguments on both sides of this issue by people that are dedicated to lofty goals. But you need to know whom you are dealing with and be especially aware of people that sell remedies they know little about. These people are only marketers, not healthcare professionals. To them, you are just a customer, not a patient, and they are happily riding on the coattails of the alternative care movement. Many alternative health providers disavow them and regard them as frauds.

There is another point to consider: many healthcare professionals will look at a scleroderma patient only through the eyes of what their specialty can provide, even though scleroderma can easily overlap many specialties. It's a big worry to many that an alternative care provider, such as a chiropractor, herbalist, or message therapist might make representations to a scleroderma patient that go completely beyond the bounds of their specialty.

I know from my past days of lurking on the Internet, it was not unusual to have a patient recount how an alternative care provider said they could help cure their scleroderma. Maybe some did get the help they needed. I'm not opposed to alternative therapies. In fact, I believe in the right of the patient to have a choice. But I am opposed to providers that misrepresent themselves, who do not have substantial experience with the specific type of involvement that a scleroderma patient has, or who refuse to work with the patient's own MD.

This book tries to give a balanced view of all sides and issues. But you need to know how to judge the value of treatment any provider offers and how to spot those that sell phony remedies, because there is nothing worse than selling snake oil to sick and desperate people.

With that being said, alternative healthcare providers can, if you choose, give you additional options and be an important part of your total care. And just like the rest of the population, scleroderma patients have differing opinions on the use of alternative treatments. Some patients are proactive from the first day of diagnosis and jump right in. Others seem to do nothing and don't even know much about the disease. In any case, patient involvement, and patient interest in alternative care can go from one extreme to the other, with most of us somewhere in the middle.

Many doctors worry about scleroderma patients using alternative therapies. They are concerned about patients self-medicating themselves and having adverse interactions; some think it is cruel to raise false hope—and others think it's just a waste of time and money.

So why do some patients leave the safety of mainstream medicine for the unchartered waters of alternative medicine? Probably because they are not getting what they want from their doctor. Doctors don't always have the answers. And it's not always a cure that patients are looking for either. Often it is the smaller problems, like healing an ulcer.

There are two key points before we continue. First, alternative care is not a replacement for conventional medicine. Second, never use alternative treatment that your doctor is unaware of. Make sure that all your healthcare providers are working together. If each knows what the other is doing, they become part of your safety net.

If you want to use alternative care providers, and if you have the right doctor, he or she will understand your need and work with you. If he or she can't, or doesn't want to, then maybe you have the wrong doctor; get a new one. If you can't find a doctor to manage your case the way you want, maybe it is a red flag—indicating that you are in dangerous territory, without a safety net.

This chapter is going to tell you what alternative medicine is and how the lines between mainstream and alternative medicine are blurring, integrating the two together, in what some hope will be the best of both worlds.

But most of all, this chapter will inform you so you can evaluate and find the right practitioners. It makes no judgments and does not encourage or discourage any treatments. But it does recognize the fact that patients often need more than what a mainstream doctor can provide. At the same time, you must recognize that by using alternative treatments, it places a far greater burden of responsibility on you; you can't afford to pick an alternative treatment the way that some people pick a diet-of-the-week. If you choose to go into these waters, this chapter will help you to stay afloat, explain the importance of involving your doctor, and hopefully maximize the potential benefits.

Who Are Alternative Care Providers?

It's important to check the credentials of a mainstream medical doctor—it is even more important to check the credentials and experience of an alternative care provider because of the lack of national standards. The first thing to look for is the initial after the name. You know that MD refers to a medical doctor who has completed four years of undergraduate college, four years of medical school, and usually two to twelve years of a medical specialty. In alternative health, you will find initials that you may not be familiar with, like DC, DO, ND and OMD. The following list describes the most common alternative specialties, educational requirements and any regulatory requirements that apply.

Chiropractor (DC)

A chiropractor is the most popular alternative health provider and is generally accepted by mainstream medical doctors and covered by many healthcare insurance policies. The profession was founded in the 1890's by an Iowa grocer and mystic healer. Today it has evolved by analyzing X-rays and palpations. Chiropractors have to be licensed under the laws of the state they practice.[82] A chiropractor looks for irregularities or misaligned vertebrae that may interfere with nerve function, and manually manipulates the spine to correct the problem. Many medical doctors tend to view chiropractors as part of mainstream treatment but consider spinal manipulation to treat a diagnosis of scleroderma as practicing in an unproved, alternative fashion.

Doctors of Oriental Medicine (OMD or DOM).

Oriental medicine is based on the belief in a vital life force said to flow through the body, and the need for a balance (yin-yang). Practitioners might be certified in all aspects of oriental medicine, or just a couple, such as acupuncture or herbal treatment.[83 84] Without investigating on your own, there is no immediate way of knowing how much education and training a practitioner has. Each state has different requirements. Acupuncturists are required to be licensed separately in thirty-four states. Some states have no licensing requirements for any part of oriental medicine. It's important to use someone who has experience with scleroderma. Read certificates and diplomas on the wall carefully, and check with your home state health-licensing agency.

Homeopathy (H)

Homeopathy was founded in the late 18th century by a German physician. It is based upon the "Law of Similars," in which the patient is treated with an extremely diluted liquid that cause symptoms similar to those the patient is experiencing. Homeopathy is almost the exact opposite of mainstream medicine because it looks for cures through the study of symptoms rather than looking for probable causes.

It is practiced by people with a wide range of backgrounds, from medical doctors to lay practitioners. There are no national standards or licenses required.[85] [86]

Naturopathic Medicine (ND)

Naturopathic Medicine can combine several alternative treatments, such as botanical medicine, nutritional therapies, homeopathy, acupuncture, hydrotherapy, Asian medicine and manipulation of muscles and bones. Medical doctors, doctors of osteopathy (DO), and doctors of chiropractic (DC) can all be trained in naturopathic medicine (and it is possible to find a provider that practices several alternative therapies), but Naturopathic Medicine is licensed and regulated in only eleven states. There are also many self-educated lay people that practice Naturopathic Medicine. The organization's website indicates no authority over national standards.[87]

The Growth Of Alternative Care

From aromatherapy[88] to vitamin therapy, 70 percent of Americans have tried, or are currently using, at least one of eight selected alternative medicines and, under the right circumstances, may be willing to try even more.

According to one survey,[89] the most popular alternative remedy is "faith healing," also known as prayer, practiced by 44 percent of the general public. Chiropractic treatment or massage found favor with 33 percent of the population, and herbal/vitamin therapy was practiced by 26 percent of Americans. Aromatherapy represented 7 percent; acupuncture or acupressure 5 percent; reflexology 5 percent; magnetic therapy 4 percent; and hypnosis 3 percent.

For most of the categories, women dominate the use of alternative medicine. The widest gender gap is in the aromatherapy category, where 12 percent of women use it versus 2 percent for men. Women also favored prayer by 51 percent versus 36 percent, and herbal/vitamin therapy 32 percent versus 19 percent.

One industry publication[90] estimated that of the $1.1 trillion spent by U.S. consumers on healthcare, $29.3 billion of the out-of-pocket expenses (deductibles and co-pays) was spent on medical doctors, compared to $34.4 billion on alternative therapies. It was further stated that visits to alternative practitioners increased from 427 million visits in 1991, to 629 million in 1997, thus exceeding total visits to all U.S. primary care physicians. It was estimated that 42 percent of alternative therapies were used exclusively to treat existing illness, and 58 percent were used, at least in part, to prevent illness or to maintain health.

Disapproving Doctors

The problem that many mainstream doctors face regarding alternative therapies is that there is not yet an authoritative source that validates the effectiveness and safety of anything but a small portion of the treatments that are out there. At this time, HerbMed[91] is one of the best sources available for consumers, but it is minuscule in size compared MEDLINE,[92] a mainstream medical database that goes back to 1966, consisting of nine million records and scientific studies that have been peer-reviewed. Although there are efforts underway to increase the number of scientific, peer-reviewed alternative remedies, there is a very long way to go to anything having the stature of MEDLINE.

Evidence-Based Medicine (EBM)

Many of today's mainstream doctors subscribe to the theory, if not practice, of evidence-based medicine (EBM).[93] In part, it calls for a process of finding controlled clinical trials of therapies that can be applied to a particular patient. It employs the practice of using scientific medical data that can be replicated.

The strict use of EBM is at somewhat of a disadvantage in treating scleroderma because it seems better oriented to a narrow search based on one symptom, not necessarily to a cluster of the interrelated symptoms that are often found in scleroderma. Of course doctors use their clinical skills and experience in treating scleroderma patients, but that can often become an exercise in trial and error, rather than an example of EBM.

Mainstream Pitfalls

Comparing mainstream to alternative therapies is not as clear-cut as some would think. Most doctors would agree that medical practice is not only based on science, but an art form as well. According to Dr. Gregg Meyer, Director of the Center for Quality Improvement and Patient Safety at the Agency for Healthcare Research and Quality, 80 percent of a doctor's work is not based on evidence.[94] Much of what doctors do is based on opinion and consensus.

The Influence of Advertising

Sometimes consensus is influenced by public opinion that is created by the advertising of new treatments, tests, drugs and devices. It can influence doctor-patient decisions, thus creating demand. A sixty second commercial on television advertising a new drug, or a twenty second spot on Oprah, can create more patient demand than the results of a carefully done clinical trial reported in the New England Journal of Medicine.[95] Hype and promotion grab the headlines and can affect medical judgment.

Drug manufactures spent $2.5 billion in 2000 on direct-to-consumer media advertising, according to IMS Health,[96] a health research firm. Pharmacists filled more than 3 billion prescriptions valued at $145 billion in 2000, up from 2 billion prescriptions valued at $65 billion in 1990.

The line between drug research and advertising has also become blurred. According to a Wall Street Journal article,[97] editors of some of the world's top medical journals are alarmed by the amount of influence drug companies have in interpreting clinical trial results on their future products. It is feared that the drug companies are using these trials as a marketing tool rather than unbiased research. Tighter standards are being considered so that the authors of these studies have control over the research, not the drug companies.

As doctors become more reliant on drugs, *pill-overload* is also becoming a very serious problem. According to a Wall Street Journal report,[98] annually there are 600,000 hospital admissions and 700,000 ER visits that were a result of medications that were taken as prescribed, but nonetheless produced side effects that required hospital care.

Combining mainstream pill-overload with alternative medicines, especially when a doctor is not aware of what a scleroderma patient is taking, creates a very dangerous situation. According to the same article, it is believed that one in five individuals who are taking prescription medications is also taking herbs, high dose vitamin supplements, or both. The solution for doctors is to end their *don't ask and don't tell* attitude concerning patients that are using alternative medicine, and to get involved.

Placebos—Pros & Cons

Taking charge of your medical care gives you more control and can create hope. Hope can sometimes be the most effective therapy you can get. Aside from possible physical benefits, alternative treatments have been known to create physiological changes in the brain that can positively affect your condition.

Some doctors would attribute this to a *placebo* effect. Most of us equate a placebo effect with a sugar pill that tricks your brain into thinking you're taking something that works. Some physicians discredit the usefulness of an alternative treatment as being no more than a placebo. On the flip-side, some alternative providers tout this as proof of the power of the mind over the body.

What causes the placebo effect? There are many studies on the subject, and just as many opinions. In general terms, it is a conditioned reflex, similar to the work done by Pavlov over one hundred years ago. But in May of 2001, a new study[99] conducted by Danish researchers even questioned the existence of the placebo effect.

On the other side, in mainstream medicine, placebos are vital in measuring a drug's effectiveness. During clinical trials, drugs are required to show they perform better than these placebo "dummies," and that the drug is not only safe and effective, but that it works in a statistically significant number of people better than a placebo or the accepted standard treatment. Vitamins, herbs and other supplements often are not held to the same standard, at least not yet.

The status of the placebo will probably continue, not only as a cornerstone in clinical drug trials, but also to be used by some mainstream doctors to discredit the effectiveness of alternative therapies.

Uninformed Medical Consumers

Some worry about the ability of the average person to understand the pitfalls of alternative treatments. According to a 1999 report in the Journal of the American Medical Association, nearly 90 million Americans, or roughly 46 percent of the adult population, are functionally illiterate when it comes to dealing with the conventional health care system.

This low health care literacy means many can't read directions written on prescription bottles, don't have a clue about what's contained in informed consent documents, don't adhere to regimens for chronic illnesses, fail to return for needed follow-up care, and don't make the necessary preparations for complicated diagnostic procedures because they misunderstand written instructions. If so many don't understand mainstream medical information and directions, the addition of alternative therapies can create an even greater danger.

Yet alternative medicine continues to grow at the expense of standard medical care. What is the source of this declining confidence? Is alternative medicine responsible for it? Is it the change in the doctor-patient relationship that resulted from the implementation of managed care, or is it just that patients want more than what is possible with mainstream medicine?

According to one industry source,[100] there are five reasons why the time-honored voice of mainstream medicine has diminished. The rise of managed care, real-time news, web-based information, a growing respect for alternatives (complementary medicine), and scientific discovery.

For scleroderma patients, it is vitally important that they feel they are helping themselves get better. If their doctor has done all that can be done without meeting the expectations of the patient, then it is likely that many will look elsewhere.

If a scleroderma patient uses an alternative therapy and sees results, it does nothing to reconcile the controversy: the patient becomes a believer, while some doctors might say that the disease had been "flaring" and coincidentally happened to go into a less active phase during the alternative treatment. The bottom line is that most scleroderma patients don't really care how it happens; they just want to get better.

Best of Both Worlds?

There are growing indications that maybe the differences between traditional and alternative medicine are not irreconcilable after all. There is a desire for many to have the best of both worlds. This trend is being fueled by the belief that doctors can't properly treat their patients who are getting alternative treatment elsewhere without becoming more knowledgeable themselves. New terms, such as "Integrative Medicine" and "Complementary Medicine" have sprung up, with "Complementary and Alternative Medicine" (CAM) becoming the most prominent.[101]

Perhaps some of this melding is based on the fact that conventional medicine is very good at fixing broken bones but does not do as good a job in dealing with degenerative diseases. It is hoped that combining mainstream and CAM will live up to a new promise of not sacrificing one for the other.

Interestingly, this integration seems to be coming more from trained medical doctors and they tend to evaluate alternative remedies the same way they evaluate traditional ones. Some mainstream organizations have even published books that evaluate alternative therapies. The Arthritis Foundation, as an example, has published one that can be very useful for scleroderma patients.[102] CAM may not attract many of the patients that are looking for a cure-in-a-bottle, but it should broaden the appeal to mainstream patients.

The White House Commission on Complementary and Alternative Medicine Policy was established in March 2000.[103] In carrying out its mandate, the Commission addresses such issues as coordinated research on complementary and alternative medical practices and products. It also is studying appropriate education and training for complementary and alternative medicine providers and traditional healthcare physicians. Another focus of the commission is the dissemination of reliable information to healthcare professionals and the general public.

The National Center for Complementary and Alternative Medicine[104] was recently given almost $90 million by Congress to study the usefulness of such popular non-traditional remedies as acupuncture, food supplements, homeopathy and body manipulation. The focus of these studies is to look for treatments that are of the greatest public health importance.

In another effort to integrate mainstream with alternative, 600 Chinese physicians and medical specialists met in June of 2001 with U.S. counterparts. The conference was sponsored by a Harvard Medical School nonprofit affiliate and focused on the two nation's health care systems and the relationship between "alternative" and "scientific" medicine. Both countries are trying to figure out how to integrate alternative medicine and scientific medicine. [105]

Further evidence of this was seen in the International Scientific Conference on Complementary, Alternative and Integrative Medicine Research, held in San Francisco in May of 2001. It provided those involved in alternative medicine with the opportunity to present research papers for review. Harvard and the University of California at San Francisco sponsored the event.

Medical schools are also getting involved. The University of Arizona was one of the first schools to start an integrative medicine program. Founded in 1994, it now includes a month-long rotation for medical students that expose them to nontraditional practices. Tucson is a hotbed for the alternative and integrative medicine movement and also home of author-physician Dr. Andrew Weil.

Harvard Medical School, acknowledging that patients are increasingly experimenting with holistic and other alternative treatments, is creating an institute for nontraditional medicine. Harvard researchers will examine the effectiveness of various treatments and will look at how they work or interact with traditional medicine.

Chapter 5

Finding Your Own Answers

This book started off by saying that it *doesn't have all the answers.* Even so, getting and using information is one of the keys to finding your *own* answers. In order to zero-in on the information you need, you need to know what your resources are and how to use them.

This chapter takes you beyond the resources that have already been noted in this book. From here, we explore how to find your own information and evaluate its worth. It's not the stuff you find in libraries; it's the *Internet*, where the only thing you have to protect yourself from bad information is your own good judgment. If you are wise in its use, the Internet can be a valuable resource that can help you micromanage this incredibly individualized disease.

The real challenge of the Internet is in filtering out the good health information from the bad. The problem of determining the value of health-related information is not limited to the Internet. But because the Internet brings you so much more, the problem of filtering and using good information is compounded many times over.

As pointed out in Chapter 4, information on the Internet is not a substitute for a face-to-face doctor-patient relationship. There is a fear by many within the scleroderma community that the inability of some patients to decipher medical information or determine what is a trustworthy source may result in doing themselves harm. I worry about it too; however, I also believe that patients have a right to be as informed and involved in their health care as they want.

It's actually very simple to stay out of harms way on the Internet. As stated before, the answer is to consult with your doctor. The root of the problem is not so much in receiving unfiltered information, but what you do with it. We are not doctors, and anyone that does not get the advice of his or her doctor before acting upon information from the Internet is at risk.

But you have to have the right doctor; if you are interested in complimentary medicine, your doctor should be able to support you. If your physician warns you of the dangers of a particular alternative remedy, you need to listen. Your doctor is your safety net.

Ten years ago, newly diagnosed scleroderma patients were faced with *limited* information that was often incomplete, outdated and sometimes inaccurate. Today, newly diagnosed patients can get an *unlimited* supply of information from the Internet that is often incomplete, outdated and sometimes inaccurate. The Internet makes much more information available, but you have to sift through so much more to determine what is useful.

How to Judge the Validity of Information

When looking for information on the Internet, search engines don't discriminate between sites that have accurate information versus inaccurate; proven treatments versus unproven. So how do you know what information to trust?

There are some simple rules to follow when getting information from the Internet. Usually, the information you need to evaluate a site is contained on the website itself. You need to look for a website's "transparency," meaning you should be able to clearly *see* enough source information so you can evaluate it. Examples would be, who owns the site, the source of the information, and if there are any potential conflicts of interest with the content provider. Generally speaking, there are four classifications of websites:

- *Dot-coms* tend to be commercial in nature. Often times, they try to sway opinion or market a service or product. But these sites could be for public service and provide public information, as well. You need to understand that, if it is a business, their profit motives may not be in your best healthcare interest.

- *Dot-orgs* are often times nonprofit organizations; they are less likely to want to sell you products or services, but can represent an organization that is trying to market or further its cause, which may not be compatible with your needs.

- *Dot-edus* usually refers to educational institutions. It does not indicate an institution's quality or reputation though. Generally, these sites do not sell products; they provide information of an academic nature.

- *Dot-gov* is reserved for federal, state, and local government. It is information that government agencies feel confident to have on its websites.

If you want to be completely safe and never expose yourself to anything that isn't proven, it might be best to stay off the Internet completely. For many though, this isn't an option because it limits their opportunity to be informed and be a full partner in their own care. Some might take the middle-road, by just venturing out to the sites of organizations that they feel have good reputations. This is a safe route to take, but others object to such a conservative approach because it prevents them from finding useful information that needs to be carefully sifted through. Whether you venture into the Internet a little or a lot, you will always need to personally evaluate and screen the material.

No single website will give you everything you're looking for. Look only as far and as deep as you're comfortable for Internet information. The following is what a *transparent* website needs to show you so you can evaluate it. If it doesn't have this most *basic* information, you can't evaluate it—be skeptical, or even discard it as a source.

What to look for
- *Who sponsors the website?*
Who owns it? You should be able to find this information in a section called *"About Us,"* or *"Who We Are."* The organization's name, address, phone number, and other contact information should be listed.

- *What is the objective of the website?*
Is it trying to sell something, directly or indirectly, or trying to change your mind? Is it academic, professional, or a public service? The objective of a website is often found under "Mission," "Our Goal," or "Purpose."

- ***Is it information or advertising?***

Does the site have advertising? Are there pop-up banners and logos of commercial companies? Does the site endorse doctors, treatments, or products? Are endorsements paid for?

- ***Is there a conflict of interest?***

Does a person or organization have a financial incentive or gain by providing the information? Does the site accept ads from companies that could influence the content of the website? Look for any possible conflict of interest.

- ***Can information be verified?***

The more authoritative the source, the more reason for confidence. Medical information should provide supporting evidence. Has it been published and is it peer-reviewed by experts? When was it published and is the information current?

If a website requires that you register, look at the site's privacy policy. What can the site do with the information you are providing? Use it to try and sell you something in the future? Sell the information to other organizations? Search the site to see if it publishes its advertising policy, or what the process is and how another organization can be linked.

Internet companies have broken their own privacy policies in the past so the safest assumption to make on your part is that registration information will be used in some way to market a product or service to you later. This isn't necessarily bad, but you must accept this if you are to proceed on such a site.

Who Do You Trust?

Trying to find good dependable health information on the web is critical. Several organizations are in the process of establishing their own "seal of approval" which will presumably make a website more transparent and easier to answer questions of authority and who provided the content.

The California HealthCare Foundation commissioned the RAND Corporation (Rand Health) to design and conduct a comprehensive study to describe and evaluate health information available on the Internet. In May of 2001, a report on the quality of health information on the Internet was published.[106] This report provides you with a detailed look at the common pitfalls of getting information from the Internet.

URAC (also known as the American Accreditation Healthcare Commission)[107] is a non-profit charitable organization representing employers, consumers, regulators, and healthcare providers of the managed care industry. In July 2001, the organization established a "seal of approval"[108] for health websites. It's an effort for the online health industry to police itself, help consumers evaluate information, and provide a forum for reporting misinformation and privacy violations. It establishes guidelines for advertising, privacy policies, and reliability of information. Sites are audited for compliance. In December of 2001, they issued their first accreditations.

Keep in mind that just because a website has one of these *seals* does not guarantee that it provides only safe and proven information. What it does do, though, is to put the privacy policy, source of information, and advertising policy in plain view. It is up to you to read these policies and evaluate the information.

Buyer Beware

Of the more than 100 million Americans using the Internet, 55 percent use it for health information, according to one source.[109] Of those that use it for health information, almost two-thirds said they don't know who provided the information, whether it could be verified, or even if the site was commercial, nonprofit, academic or government sponsored.

Beware of any site that is selling something using one of the following claims:

- Sells through glowing testimonials.
- Claims the product is "natural" and "nontoxic" (implying no side affects).
- An ancient remedy.
- Claims it is an effective "cure."
- Claims of a "money-back" guarantee.
- Failure to list supporting evidence of its claims.
- Claims that the product is available from only one source.
- Failure to list the company's name, address, phone number or other contact information.

In response to the growing problem of health scams on the Internet, in June of 2001 the FTC and FDA cracked down on Internet quackery. Their first target were sites selling colloidal silver. It's a substance that many sites claim can cure acne, herpes, cancer, leprosy and the bubonic plague, plus more than 650 different disease-causing viruses. Not to be excluded are the additional claims that it gives the body "a superior second immune system," and has Viagra-like power to spice up your sex life.

CyberDocs may be bad for your health

"CyberDocs" offering medical consultations via the Internet are not necessarily qualified, and some may be dispensing "dubious health advice," according to a letter published in the November 7, 2001 issue of The Lancet,[110] a medical journal in the UK. "Patients should be warned that there are currently no means to determine the credibility or qualification of cyberdocs on the Internet," the researchers write. On the other side, there are organizations, such as QuackWatch,[111] that are trying to let consumers know about medical misinformation.

Surfing the Web

The Internet is disorderly; it's not like going to a library to find a book; you don't have the use of a librarian and you're on your own. In addition, there is no card catalog to find what you need, and no such thing as a comprehensive search. It is often like trying to find a needle in a haystack. This chapter assumes that you have had some experience in many of the Internet basics. Overviews and resources are provided, but this is not a tutorial on the Internet's finer points.

It is also assumed that you have some familiarity with search engines. Though many of us are unaware of how the various search engines work, there are differences between them. Some are based on subject catalogs, loosely based on how a traditional library is set up. Others strictly use key words to search for any document that contains those words. With most search engines, the order of your keywords can also affect your results.

Regardless of which search engines you use—and it is recommended that you use two or three for a good search, you will probably never get the same results twice. Often times, the results will be different, even on the same search engine from one time to the next. You should also be aware that the order in which the first hits appear might be influenced by advertising dollars.

How To Surf

The more you know about what information you are looking for, the greater the chance of a successful search. If you are only looking for information on scleroderma, it makes for a relatively easy search because you are not going to come up with that much information on a standard search engine. As an example, a search of *diabetes* might yield a couple of thousand *hits* on a typical search engine,[112] *scleroderma* might only produce a few dozen.

If you are looking for information on specific issues, your search becomes more complicated. For example, when looking for resources on how a family can cope with scleroderma, the results will depend upon your method of search. Using the keywords of *family-coping-disease* to search, you will probably end up with many sites that refer to coping with specific diseases. Delete coping and just search *family-disease*, you'll notice a few new sites popped up that are national and local support organizations for patients and families that are not specific to any disease. There is no single way to do this. Experiment and play around with your search words.

There are some general rules to keep in mind when searching. We are not going to go into detail about the intricacies of each engine, but keep in mind that with some, you can focus your search by using what is called Boolean searches. A Boolean is used when you have two or more words that are separated by AND (the word on either side of AND must be contained in the document), OR (at least one of the words must be in document), NOT (will look for the first word in documents only if the second word is not present). The AND, OR, NOT must be in caps. Booleans can sometimes be essential to finding what you are looking for in the least amount of time. Booleans, if not automatically employed by the search engine, are sometimes available if there is an option for "advance search."

Hints to Pinpointing the Topic

Key words describe what is being looked for. Do words have different meanings? Are there other words that also describe it? You are sometimes better off using the rarest words first, such as *interstitial* AND *scleroderma* AND *lungs.*

Meta-Engines

A *Meta-Engine* is a search engine that uses dozens of other search engines to do their search. Google.com is an example, and will produce many more hits than a standard search engine, but may, or may not get you better results.[113]

For example, when *scleroderma* is used as a search word, it can produce over 80,000 hits. It offers a much wider array of information, from commercial to scientific developments, even bulletin board postings. It is important to remember that the search engine ranks the first hit as being what it thinks is most relevant (unless the ranking is paid for) and the last being the least, so as you work your way through them, you are likely to find hits that seem less and less relevant.

Other Sources

Aside from search engines, there is substantial Internet based information that has been cataloged by professional librarians. Although not always the best information on the disease itself, it can be an excellent way to find information on family, insurance, legal, and financial issues. A good start in finding reference resources online is the Internet Public Library.[114] Others include The Librarians' Index to the Internet,[115] and The World Wide Web Virtual Library.[116]

Tracking federal legislation—such as funding bills for autoimmune diseases and scleroderma research—can be done through Thomas, named in honor of Thomas Jefferson.[117] You can also get to this site through the Library of Congress.[118]

As you click through these sites and their related links, you will come upon other valuable resources. It can be very helpful if you bookmark and organize points of interests on these sites so you can build your own reference system and have them when you need them. Appendix B has some good ones to start with.

The U.S. National Library of Medicine is the ultimate peer-reviewed medical database. There are about 9 million records from medical journals and other authoritative sources dating back to 1966. A free searchable version of this database is available through PubMed.[119] Using Boolean searches is a good way to search a specific scleroderma topic. For example, if you only use *scleroderma* to search, as of the publishing date of this book, you will get 11,492 hits. That is not going to help much. But using the Boolean AND the *current month and year*, you can see what has been published for the current month. Or, if you know that your doctor has had something published, search *scleroderma* AND *name of doctor*. This also works well when checking the credentials of a new doctor.

If you want to know what papers have been published on lung involvement, you need to know the medical terminology your doctor uses to describe the exact condition. If you only search *scleroderma* AND *lung* you'll come up with 936 hits. *Scleroderma* AND *lung* AND *interstitial* narrows it to 219 hits. One more search word, or date, would make it manageable. You will also find that many of these hits may not be viable because they only refer to scleroderma in passing, or are outdated. Maybe you've heard others talking about a just-published study; this method of search allows you to read it first hand.

You're not a doctor; so what are you going to do with this information? It depends. For most of us, we will be able to educate ourselves better on a particular issue. Information from medical journals is sometimes technical but there is a surprising amount in straightforward English. If you find something you think applies to your case, take a copy of the report with you to your next doctor's appointment and discuss it.

News Databases

Valuable information about scleroderma and related issues are published in newpapers, magazines, and professional journals all the time. A lot of this can be accessed through Internet sites such as Yahoo!, but not all of it. With some, you might have to go through gated websites to get at them—and they cost money. These include Dialog, Lexis-Nexis, Dow Jones Interactive and Gale Research, just to name a few.

As an alternative to paying for these services, sometimes they can be accessed at a college library, where Internet access to these services is often free. It is even becoming more common at public libraries.

Support

There is a difference between researching the Internet for information and using it to seek the emotional support of other scleroderma patients. The web can provide excellent forums that can bring patients emotionally together. Instead of reading about information from organizations, companies and institutions, you get people's opinions—and everybody has one.

Some people are afraid that patients will confuse other people's opinions with facts; they are the ones that fear online support groups the most. The truth is, some scleroderma forums do a better job than others in distinguishing fact from opinion; you shouldn't assume that any of them are automatically doing it for you. It is ultimately your responsibility.

Newsgroups and mailing lists (sometimes referred to as digests) are two of the most popular ways to connect with other scleroderma patients. A newsgroup[120] is often unrestricted, with fewer rules than a mailing list. Anybody can read the posts, but to make your own post, registering may be required.

Mailing lists (digests)[121] are a more controlled environment. There is usually a moderator that reviews all incoming e-mails and is responsible for maintaining certain standards. You have to subscribe to a mailing list in order to participate. Messages come to you via e-mail so you don't have to go to a special site.

In addition, there are many places on the Internet, such as AOL, Yahoo!, and iVillage, that have scleroderma chat rooms and bulletin boards.

Chapter 6

A Scleroderma Family

I have always recorded what was going on in my life: what I felt, why I did things, the progress of my family, even business issues. I can't explain why—it just seemed like a natural thing for me to do.

When I was eighteen years old, I started writing in a daily journal. By the time I was nineteen, I dropped the written journal in favor of an audio journal on an old reel-to-reel tape recorder. A few years later, it migrated to cassettes and micro-cassettes, and is now being recorded in a digital format.

For thirty-four years, from college days and my first date with Karen, and throughout our marriage—kids, business, highs and lows—my audio journal continues today. It now consists of a couple thousand hours of recordings. It has provided me with a sense of where I've been, and where I'm going in life; it helps me resolve problems, and gives me clarity.

During Karen's illness, especially during the times when I felt the most alone and isolated, it was often the only thing I had in helping me to sort things out—it was incredibly therapeutic. Many of these tapes were used as a resource in writing this book.

The previous chapters of this book were not difficult to write; they were just based upon what I wanted and needed to know as Karen's disease progressed. These last two chapters deal with the personal side of how scleroderma affects the family and being a caregiver. They were much harder to write.

With these two chapters, I wanted to help patients and families with what they wanted and needed, but I couldn't initially decide how to do it. Just giving facts and resources didn't seem like enough.

Aside from protecting personal privacy, I questioned what I could offer others that would help. Every situation is different, and it seemed impossible to provide information that applied to everyone. Also, I'm not an authority, and I didn't want to preach words of wisdom, tell how inspiring and noble it is to be a caregiver (it's grossly overrated), or regurgitate what others have already said (there are already many books available).[122]

Just as each patient's medical case is unique, so is the personal side of his or her family's ordeal. Regardless of what experts say or what I have to offer, there is no universal formula that will work. No one can zero-in on the personal dynamics of each family's needs. But like the disease itself, there are some common issues; some that are generic and apply to other chronic diseases, and others that are specific to scleroderma.

With this in mind, I concluded that the best way for me to provide anything of value was to just give a personal account. Please keep in mind that my family is only one story—there are thousands of others that have not yet been told. I hope that we will all have the opportunity to read many more accounts in the future (see Appendix A).

As is the case with all families, my family is unique. In addition, the severity and speed of Karen's case compressed and even distorted what others might experience. But I believe that many of the issues that are addressed in the next two chapters will resonate with most scleroderma families. Learning things the hard way is called experience: learning from other peoples' mistakes is called wisdom. Any insights you get from my account will probably be as much from my mistakes as from what I did right. I hope you will be able to leap past some of my flaws and gain some wisdom of your own.

Maybe the biggest value in reading someone else's account is that you can see that others feel many of the same things you do; it helps legitimize your feelings and accept them as being normal. Even though it doesn't provide all the answers, just like support groups and the virtual online support community, hearing the stories of others reminds us that we are not alone—and that can help a lot.

Karen—Before SD

It would have been hard to imagine a married couple being more different than Karen and me.

She was outgoing, I'm introspective; she was intuitive, I'm analytical; she was spontaneous, I ponder; she was suggestive, I'm contrary; she lived for the day, I plan for tomorrow; she worried about what others would think, I focus on results.

Karen was born in New York in 1950, and moved to Los Angeles with her parents, older brother and sister, when she was two years old. Typical of the time, her mother was a homemaker; her father, a postal employee who always seemed to have a second job to help maintain their modest home. Her world took an abrupt turn when her father died of cancer when she was eight years old. She watched her unprepared mother shoulder the burden of suddenly having to work and support the family.

It left her with a need to be self-reliant and a desire to make her own "mark" in life. She had a natural gift for being able to inspire and motivate people with her enthusiasm. Until she was diagnosed with scleroderma in 1998, she dedicated much of her life to being the ultimate volunteer for charities, both big and small.

Karen defined herself by her desire to touch the lives of other people. She took great pleasure in communicating and socializing with any—and everybody. In part, her self-image had not only to do with her appearance, but her boundless energy, and a can-do spirit in working with people. It put her center stage, and brought out the best in her. It was a perfect fit in helping to make her "mark" in life, one person at a time.

I loved her charm, admired her spunk, and respected her grit. She was the master of her own life, and her personal sense of giving made her a favorite confidant. Though we were both strong-willed in what we wanted, I tended to accept things I thought were beyond my control. It usually never occurred to her that something was beyond her control: she just got what she wanted.

Karen was the family glue, and as she got older, she just got better. She looked forward to the future—until scleroderma blew it out the window.

Me—Before SD

I was born in a Los Angeles suburb in 1948. My father was an engineer, my mother, even though working on-and-off throughout my childhood, somehow always conveyed the impression that she was a full-time homemaker. Though I don't remember being particularly happy as a kid, it never occurred to me that my childhood was anything less than perfect, if not a bit boring.

I describe myself as being cynically optimistic; I tend to look on the positive side of life, but try not to be too stupid about it. Being negative seems like a waste of time and energy. It has always been important for me to do the best I can. Much of my motivation in life is based upon the realization that I am going to be dead far longer than alive, and I want to make the most of it.

Karen loved being with people; it made me socially lazy—not that I would have been much different without her. I never had to think about our social plans; she did it all, and that was fine with me. It even gave me the luxury of being more direct with people than many were comfortable with—I always knew that Karen would offset my shortcomings and people would probably continue to put up with me.

Watching Karen in a room full of people, as each one knew that she was there just for them, was poetry for me. Nothing would have made me happier than to continue to sit back and be a part of her magic for the rest of my life.

The Diagnosis

Karen didn't have to endure years, or even months, of not knowing what the diagnosis was; she didn't have to suffer the innuendos of other people questioning that something was really wrong. However, even though her diagnosis came quickly, thus validating that there was a diagnostic *label* that could be put on her condition, there was a few weeks when she did not know for sure. It put her in a state of extreme anxiety. Having always been in control of her life, she could not stand the uncertainty, even for a short time.

During this time, she told some friends in hushed tones *something was wrong*. From the beginning, the likely suspect was scleroderma. Her first information about the disease came mostly by word-of-mouth—someone who knew someone who had it, or friends that had read something about it. None of this gave a clear picture of the disease, and, in fact, it confused and scared her. One friend said that she heard of a woman who had it for many years and her main complaint was that she could no longer go windsurfing. I thought at the time, "maybe this isn't so bad" after all—Karen didn't windsurf. One comment from an acquaintance left Karen in disbelief when the woman enviously said, "maybe your breasts will get firmer."

On the other hand, others reported that the disease was very disfiguring, especially in the face. This terrified her. She had also heard of how it could kill by attacking the internal organs—she flippantly passed it off as being preferable to disfigurement.

She knew that she was not the first, or the only one, facing the prospect of scleroderma. Some must surely have been worse off than she, others better. Nevertheless, neither of us were able to think of anyone else—the thought of the disease was all consuming. Even before all the symptoms appeared, she was totally preoccupied with the disease. We could only focus on our own personal catastrophe and felt we were alone in a cold and very uncaring world.

We didn't know what lay ahead, but we did sense that life, as we knew it, ended even before the diagnosis.

After the Diagnosis

Due to the unpredictable nature of scleroderma, Karen's anxiety level did not decrease after the diagnosis. In fact, it just created more uncertainty.

Karen always felt that life had a grand plan for her—and scleroderma wasn't it. She had always been in control of her life. This disease was not only a physical danger to her; scleroderma threatened to take away her very identity, and left her with no power to do anything about it.

She was obsessed with knowing how or why this happened. All kinds of thoughts raced through her mind. She knew that something had seriously gone wrong, and she wanted answers. She felt the need to identify the culprit.

Even if she had been able to find out how this happened, she figured it still had to be a mistake. If it wasn't a mistake, then this must be some type of punishment for something she did . . .but what? What could she have done to deserve this? She also dwelled on the possibility that she had come into contact with some kind of toxic substance that had triggered it.

Experts that deal with how to cope with chronic illnesses could easily put labels on each of her feelings. They weren't unique, and you didn't have to be an expert to see her denial and anger. I read over one hundred books during her illness, several of which dealt with coping with a chronic disease. I learned a lot about this *process*. None really gave me what I wanted (which was to make things the way they were before), but they did help by putting our situation into perspective.

Eighty percent of the physical damage scleroderma inflicted upon Karen occurred within the first ten months. It seemed like a downhill-only roller coaster ride. There never seemed time to catch her breath or to adjust to these radical changes. Denial rapidly gave way to anger and frustration. She looked at herself as damaged goods. Her loss of independence made her feel like she had to ask permission to do everything. She lost her dignity. She saw herself as a mannequin, or a rag doll, that others just picked up and put where they wanted. She turned her quick wit on herself, inflicting a type of gallows humor, chiding and making fun of herself.

During this time, the durable medical equipment started to arrive. It was everywhere in the house; it became so common that the rest of the family just treated it like furniture. Karen hated all of it. Instead of looking at it as being able to help her adapt to her condition, the equipment became a symbol of the disease. She said that if the equipment couldn't give her back her old life, it was of no use to her.

Her personality also changed. She went from feeling like she was on the stage of life, to a circus sideshow, or even worse—invisible. She felt as though she had lost her old identity that she was once so proud of. She was unable to tell the difference between her new identity and the disease. To her, it had become one and the same. During the first few months, she cried uncontrollably several times a day.

As her facial features became affected, the reduced movement in her jaw and tongue, plus the reduced lung function dealt her one of the cruelest blows of all: the loss of much of her communication skills. Shopping in stores, once a favorite pastime became a nightmare. Clerks were unable to hear her, and some shoppers were oblivious, bumping and tripping over her wheelchair. Others just stared. Sometimes it made her so uncomfortable and depressed that she avoided public places altogether.

She was afraid that her appearance would eventually get so bad that she would scare children (this never happened). Ironically, many years before, Karen had found it very difficult to be around people with certain types of disabilities and deformities. However, her involvement with a charity that represented many children in wheelchairs forced her to confront her fears, and she eventually found that her compassion was stronger than the fear, and it just stopped being an issue.

She dwelled on how guilty she felt (about everything), from what she was doing to me and the kids, to even berating herself for refusing to have life insurance.

In addition, even though she felt the disease had already stripped her of her life, scleroderma still wasn't finished with her—it just continued to march on, constantly finding new ways to show its power over her; there never seemed to be a rock bottom to this disease. Even if it did quiet down for a while, when a new symptom appeared, it would re-ignite the whole cycle of fear and anger all over again.

The uncertainty terrified her, never knowing where scleroderma would strike next. She periodically had "brain fog," and was unable to think clearly. Aside from forgetfulness, she was unable to distinguish minor side affects from major problems. She even began to wish that she had a more straightforward disease, like cancer, where you get chemotherapy, and you either make it or you don't. She was often in a profound state of depression.

Along with the denial, anger, fear and frustration, Karen, as well as the entire family, experienced a type of chronic grief. At different times and in different ways, each of us grieved, as though we were mourning the loss of the *old* Karen. Each of us related to it a little bit differently.

For Karen, it was the recognition that she lost the simple sweetness of life that she had always taken for granted, and for the things she knew she would never have. She never failed to look, even if she didn't say anything, at an older couple that was happily walking hand-in-hand; or at a friend's new grandchild. Sometimes she would just stare from her bed into her open closet, looking, but not able to see any of her old clothes she could still wear. (I never got rid of any of her old clothes, even though our three daughters made us closet poor. I hoped the old clothes would be some sort of incentive for her. Besides, if I moved them, I was afraid it would be a sign to her that I had given up.) As a result, fashion-less, easy-to-wash clothes with elastic waistbands were squeezing her old clothes out. For her, the *old* Karen was gone, and what remained she didn't recognize.

Kids

Before scleroderma, Karen was the dominant force in our kids' lives. She was personal confidant and advisor, social and fashion consultant. After her diagnosis, she could no longer play the full role (and sometimes none at all). It was very wounding for her not to be able to fully respond to her mothering instincts.

During Karen's illness, our three daughters all lived at home. Their ages ranged from early teens to early twenties. Early on, when it was obvious that something was wrong, but before her diagnosis, they all treated it like it was the flu: here today, maybe gone by tomorrow; never a thought that anything could happen to their Mom.

Even after the diagnosis, the kids seemed only able to look at Karen's disease in the present tense. Initially, I thought that was okay, because the unpredictability of scleroderma made it difficult to give a picture of what the future might be. But even though they saw her rapid deterioration before their very eyes, on almost any given day, they never gave much of an impression that the future would be different than that day.

Karen had the view that her identity was suddenly taken away from her. She was very hard on herself because she had never done anything at less than 100 percent. Doing less was never acceptable: not 50 percent, not 70 percent, or even 90 percent. For Karen, it was all or nothing.

Our kids had a different perspective. They instinctively knew she couldn't do and be everything she was before. They all accepted this, I thought, with amazing resilience and grace. Even though they saw what the disease had done to her, they didn't see Karen as being physically or emotionally disabled from being their Mom. I think that may have been because they saw that she was still giving 100 percent of what she had left.

As the disease progressed, we wanted to have them know as much about her condition as they wanted to know, but didn't want to over-burden any of them and force more information than they could handle. I assumed that what they could handle had a lot to do with their ages. Two of them were young adults, and I had greater expectations of what they could deal with compared to the youngest. As it turned out though, their individual personalities and characters had as much to do with what they wanted to know as their age. Typically, one daughter didn't want the details, only my assurance that Karen wouldn't die (which I said I didn't know). Another wanted every little bit of medical detail but shielded her feelings. And the third just accepted what was good and ignored everything else as best she could.

As time passed, I did talk with each one individually. I took great pains to be very clear, and confirmed what I thought had to be obvious: Karen was getting much worse. When asked by two of the three if she was going to die, I said that the disease would shorten her life, but that I didn't know by how much; it would probably be sooner than later.

I don't think they really ever accepted my efforts in trying to get them to see what course this disease might take. It always seemed to me like they were giving themselves a choice of whom they wanted to believe. Karen always told each of them as little girls that she wasn't going to die until she was very old and they didn't need her anymore. Mom always told better stories than Dad.

Maybe this helps explain why their individual roles within the family didn't change much either. I was expecting them to be super-sensitive, walking on eggshells, going way overboard to please. But when Karen's condition was status quo, each of their shortcomings, whether it was messiness, dodging household chores, or intolerance to something or someone, remained basically unchanged.

However, when Karen was at her worst, they did usually snap-to. They all made concerted efforts, in their own way, to make things easier for both me and Karen. Occasionally, someone, or even all of us, would crack under the weight of just plain misery. Either way though, I never got the feeling that their actions or behavior had much to do with any fear of the future; it mostly seemed in response to whatever the current circumstances were.

Our youngest daughter did get one dividend though. The older girls felt they had received the full benefits of having Karen as an active mother, and that the younger sister was getting short-changed. Independently, each tried to make up for some of that difference.

They all tended to instinctively pitch in to help maintain rituals that were important to the family: one sitting next to Karen at dinner time to help her eat so we could all eat together; family rides in the car required them to struggle, getting a wheelchair in and out of a trunk that was too small. They also knew how important Karen's appearance was to her, so one put herself in charge of makeup, another in charge of her hair.

Karen's sensory perceptions seemed to go counter to her overall physical deterioration. For some reason, just as it seemed every part of her body was failing, Karen became supersensitive to sound—as though she acquired the ears of a dog. If someone were eating two rooms away, the noise from normal chewing would drive her crazy.

When one of us went over the edge emotionally, feelings were hurt, voices raised, and doors slammed. At one time or another, each would hide away in her room for refuge. It was just a momentary respite though, because there really was no escape for anybody. The burden of scleroderma dominated and controlled every aspect of our lives—and we staggered under its weight.

Family

After the diagnosis, Karen started talking to people about the disease. It helped to unburden her. Starting with close family members, she worked her way out to friends, providing various degrees of detail.

Her side of the family's reaction was very supportive. With some, she was comfortable in speaking about every minute detail. She was able to not only talk about the medical details, but her feelings as well. In that regard, they provided a much better sounding board for her than I did. She wanted sympathy for how "unfair and unjust" the disease was, and she got it.

Friends

Karen had more friends and knew more people than anyone I ever knew. Her friends came from many places in her life, and she related to each one a little bit differently. Some she had a lot in common with. With others, she admired, but had less common ground. She met many of them through charitable work.

Initially, there was an outpouring of concern. Most thought it was serious from the beginning but, with the key words being *inflammation* and *tight skin*, were unable to anticipate what would happen. One friend later said that she equated it with a bad form of arthritis—something you just have to suffer with. She felt badly when it became apparent that she had grossly underestimated the disease.

As her condition worsened, a battery of friends came out for her, almost like they were in lock step, letting her know how much they cared. Everyone seemed to have their own way of showing their concern. Personal visits, phone calls, notes, flowers, books (and later books-on-tape) constantly arrived. One even built ramps for her wheelchair. My personal favorite was when someone brought an entire dinner to the house.

Staying in close contact with someone who has a progressive disease can emotionally wear people down. Watching Karen deteriorate was horrifying for some to witness, and increasingly depressing for others. For those that wanted to stay as close as possible, it meant that they would be unable to avoid feeling her pain and suffering.

Surprisingly, only two people that were actively visiting her from the beginning actually faded out of her life. One just couldn't take the emotional toll. After a few months, she just stopped calling or stopping by. It was too painful for her to be around Karen. She openly chastised herself by saying she had "a character defect." Another friend, after a very long time, just slowly slipped away. She continued to call but stopped coming by for visits.

Chapter 6

As the disease progressed, I usually had to tell people that she wasn't up to talking on the phone or able to see visitors. I was surprised at how persistent many of these people were. I think that if it was me calling someone in Karen's situation, I probably would have given up after a few times. I was impressed with the perseverance most of them showed.

Some of her friends came and just talked like they always did, trying their best to ignore the disease. Others found it very difficult; it was as though scleroderma had taken away their common ground. In the old days, Karen was a good listener, but if there were ever any gaps in the conversation, or where the other person was uncomfortable, Karen would make it right. Now, it was awkward for some, and without Karen's help, they didn't know what to say.

Scleroderma unavoidably changed Karen's relationship with everybody to some extent. Some thought it was their job to cheer her up. Others were clearly uncomfortable in trying to provide comfort. Some efforts backfired: if someone told her how good she looked, she felt they were invalidating how she felt. If someone would just stop by, saying they were passing by on their way someplace, Karen would feel like it was an afterthought. If someone complained about something trivial in their life, she would think of them as being insensitive.

On the other hand, others went too far the other way. They felt the enormity of what Karen was facing and felt that, in comparison, there was nothing in their life that was worth talking about. They wanted to just talk about what Karen wanted to talk about. But Karen just wanted to hear about others because it got her mind off of how she was feeling.

When she was deeply depressed or in constant pain, there was just no winning. Karen would think people didn't understand, or worse, were uncaring. She felt she always used to listen and empathize with others. Now, she wanted some of that back.

A New Status Quo

In the beginning, there was nothing normal about having scleroderma. It changed our family's structure and way of life from top to bottom. Yet we eventually had no choice but to accept its domination. Maybe it was a warped and surreal version of what we considered *normal*, but we did become accustomed to it. For Karen and me, how we adapted (or didn't adapt), to the changes the disease forced upon us had a huge impact on our ability to provide quality of life for the entire family.

Scleroderma required us to change the order of our priorities. Some things that were once important had even become irrelevant. Many of the things that we once built our material dreams upon became secondary. The trappings of money (not its utility value), and what we owned, were overshadowed by the need to emotionally stay connected and united.

Chapter 7

Caregiving

On-The-Job Training

From the beginning, even before the diagnosis was confirmed, I went with Karen to her doctor appointments and filled her prescriptions. As her condition deteriorated, I split the housework with our daughters, and did the marketing and cooking. I dressed and bathed her, and moved her from bed to wheelchair to couch and back again throughout the day and night. When the pain was more than she could bear, I massaged her hands, arms and legs for hours. It wasn't until weeks later, when a home health nurse asked who her caregiver was, that I realized—it was me. It wasn't planned—it just happened.

From the beginning, I wanted to help her as much as I could, but I had no way of understanding what *help* was going to mean. I was not sure that I had even ever heard of the term *caregiver* before. In the beginning, I didn't know what she was going to need or what I was going to be able to do; I just knew I wanted to be there for her.

Looking back, I realize that the way I defined my caregiving role had as much to do with my age and the particular point in my life that it happened, as with my own personal desire to be involved. For example, my role would have been much different if it had happened ten years earlier, when our kids were much younger and business obligations consumed me. On the other hand, if it had happened ten years later, I doubt that I would have had the physical stamina and strength to do even half of what I did. One thing is for sure though: regardless of when it might have happened, I would never have been able to anticipate what I would be facing, either emotionally or physically. It was on-the-job training.

Society and the Caregiver

It's only been in recent years that society started to consider how a spouse's illness affects the healthy care–giving spouse. Care-giving spouses have been historically over-shadowed by the patient, and even when acknowledged, were often described as saints, martyrs, stoics—and women.

Things are different today. Public awareness, education and support for the caregiver have increased dramatically.[123] In fact, services and support tend to be underutilized, if for no other reason than most caregivers are unaware that these services exist. The gap between female verses male caregivers has narrowed to 56 percent vs. 44 percent respectively, according to the National Family Caregivers Association. Though a big change, it still represents a big gap for female scleroderma patients. (Do the math: 80 percent scleroderma patients are women, 44 percent of caregivers are men.)

As unlikely and ill suited as I felt I was for being a caregiver, demographically my family and I were probably as close as any to being a typical scleroderma family.

Just as we've seen scleroderma patients become more involved in the decision-making process of their care, today's caregivers are emerging with a new perspective that sheds much of the old image. As Karen became more and more dependent upon me, I desperately looked for information on caregiving that might give me a clue as to how I could survive this new role. The following are some of the tips I found.

- Get enough rest. Fatigue is a major problem because of the need to hold down a job, and run the household, in addition to giving care.

- Ask others for help, for day-to-day tasks, or for personal time off.

- Join a support group.

- Feel your emotions and realize they're normal.

- Take charge of your life.

These guidelines sounded reasonable: if I didn't take care of myself, I would be of little use to Karen and our kids. The only problem was, I ignored these and most other tips, especially in the beginning. You'd think that if I were smart enough to research it, I would at least use it (you're giving me too much credit). In my defense, I will say, that due to the speed and severity of her case, I felt that if I followed traditional guidelines, she would not survive.

Time was of the essence. I felt she either needed a miracle, or some new medical breakthrough—and *fast*. If either of these didn't pan out, then it was up to me to find a way to save her. I didn't know how, but I was going to try. This was my state of mind at the time; I had no doubt that if someone or something didn't intervene, she would soon die.

We probably should have talked more openly about caregiving issues and my role in the very beginning, but I don't know how much good this would have done. We had no clue as to how various issues were going to play out, so I doubt that it would have made much of a difference. We never even determined if we both had similar goals for her care, we just assumed we did (we didn't). In the beginning, I put all her fears to rest by saying, "Don't worry. I'm going to get you better—whatever it takes."

And so, I started my single-minded quest to get her better. The only problem was, the more I learned about scleroderma and what I'd have to do as a caregiver, the more impossible it seemed to look.

I eventually solved the problem; the answer was so simple; I don't know why it took me so long to come up with it—I just decided to do the impossible. I would provide all the caregiving, manage all the medical issues, work more to offset rising medical costs and the loss of Karen's income, and although I didn't think I would have time to find a cure for the disease (after all, I have my limits), I was pretty sure that I could at least find a partial one for Karen. Once I had these little details out of the way, I set the groundwork to implementing a plan.

I knew I had to move fast—no time to waste (like talking about all of this with Karen). I moved all of my work into a home office and reduced business travel to a minimum so I could be with her twenty-four hours a day, (except for two or three week-long trips a year). Next, since nothing was as important to me as Karen, I had to get rid of anything in my life that diverted my attention away from her; like my own ambitions and personal comfort. (My intentions were good; I just wanted to save her.)

So how does a savior go about saving someone, you ask? I didn't have a lot of experience in this matter. My usual fallback position told me to do what I've always done when confronted by unfamiliar problems: research it and find a better way. But as you saw in the previous example, getting the right information doesn't always mean I'll use it.

Instead, I decided to build upon the folly of being a saint, martyr, and stoic. My plan was to improve upon this guaranteed formula for failure by employing what I knew best: business. To me, it was all a matter of management style. I reorganized our work force (family), created a new paradigm that would streamline and reduce all non-core activities (kids and forsaking personal kindness to others), focused totally on the needs of the customer (Karen), with maximum support on R&D, creative utilization of home infusion resources, and limit the need for radical invasive procedures (unless all else failed). For those of you that just let that blow past you, it was just a very pompous way of saying that I reacted as though I was implementing a business plan, with a mission statement, objectives and all. I think that I just had a case of too much testosterone.

Actually, in writing down the pros and cons of being a caregiver, I concluded that I was a poor candidate. I had few of the job qualifications and skill sets that were necessary. I was undomesticated, took directions poorly, and constantly questioned the opinions of experts that knew far more than me. But I was strong, ignorant, and willing. I freely applied for this mission, and was proud when I got the job—but was sorry I never got a chance to see any of the other candidates. No matter—traditional caregiving was only secondary for me; my main goal was to get my wife back.

I'm not going to give you a checklist of what to do. I'm not going to tell you where I made mistakes (unless it was a really big one); read on and you can see for yourself (they're not hiding). I'm just going to give you the story, pretty much unvarnished. Keep in mind that our case was compressed into a relatively short period of time. Also remember, my intentions were better than some of the results. I meant well, I just wanted to be her White Knight, to save her from this cruel disease.

PHASE 1

I wasn't ignorant to the fact that I couldn't indefinitely sustain my one-sided agenda. I just couldn't see an alternative. I felt boxed into a dreadful corner and could only see one lousy choice: to ignore my own feelings and put them in constant conflict with what I thought she needed. As you will see, my ideas on caregiving often didn't hold—some because they were stupid, and others because my single-minded determination made her feelings irrelevant. But I did learn a couple of things along the way—like what was most important to both of us, and how painfully sweet life could be. Unfortunately, like most other scleroderma experiences, I learned all these things the hard way. A little wisdom would have helped a lot.

From the beginning, it was important for me to believe that I had more control over the situation than was possible. I knew I was fooling myself, that this *virtual* control existed only in my own mind; but I felt I had no alternative because I didn't believe that mainstream medicine was going to be able to do enough for her. However, this kind of thinking did yield an unexpected bonus from medical professionals. I felt that doctors and nurses, and in fact, almost every healthcare professional we came in contact with, took notice of my complete dedication to Karen's care. I believe that in turn, it helped motivate each of them to give a *little extra* effort for her.

This manufactured sense of control I had also provided me with hope. It allowed me to see and recognize what I could do, and ignore what I couldn't. It forced me to keep my head down though, taking just one step at a time. It was a lot easier to just look at that next step—it might be the step that makes a difference. If I looked up to see how many steps I had to go, I would have become demoralized and gone into a state of emotional paralysis. I needed to feel that I could influence what would happen to her with my next step, otherwise, I'd be irrelevant—and I wasn't able to bear that.

In the beginning, Karen's fear of scleroderma overwhelmed her. For the first time in our marriage, she was obviously scared and vulnerable. She looked to me for help—and I didn't hesitate in wanting to be her hero. I looked upon myself as her advocate, the one that would manage everything for her: relieve her of personal responsibilities, deal with healthcare providers, and, let's not forget the most important part—to make her better. A simple plan, no?

I felt that her pain and suffering made it difficult for her to think clearly. I took it upon myself to lift the burden: I decided what she needed, and what was best for her. She accepted this at first, falling into line; she assumed the role of a traditional patient, and followed *doctor's* orders (me). She was a very good sport about it, trying to swallow dozens of alternative concoctions that I researched (and advised her doctors of). I also babied her, something we weren't used to usually doing: she liked it and found it comforting. She desperately wanted to share my vision that it was possible for her to get better.

During this time, the nights became progressively disrupted. I had always been a heavy sleeper—fast to go to sleep and hard to wake up. I got used to tuning-in and subconsciously listening for her (usually); a pain, an itch, the toilet, a bucket—whatever it was—I would immediately spring into action when awakened. Maybe *spring* isn't the right word; it was hard for me to be alert on such short notice, often tripping and falling on my way to her. Once I was awake though, especially if it was for more than fifteen minutes, my chances of going right back to sleep diminished considerably. If she were on the toilet for 5 minutes, I would doze on the bed for four.

As her condition worsened, she was horrified at the thought that I would have to take care of all her body care needs—and yet at the same, she was just as afraid that I wouldn't. It was the ultimate humiliation for her. To limit this, I took charge of all her personal care. I didn't want her to feel that she had to ask others; I didn't want others to pity her. Though this worked in the short run, it was an absolute disaster for me in the long term. It gave me no viable substitute for relief or respite. It made me not only the preferred caregiver, but as long as I was in the same county, the only acceptable one. We became tethered together, twenty-four hours a day. Thereafter, whenever Karen needed help, and I was not in the room but others were—someone would come running for me, saying "Quick! Karen needs you!"

The disease was unrelenting in its attack. Everyday seemed like something got worse and something new appeared. I thought I would be able to push back these scleroderma assaults with quick commands from the doctor's e-mails and the rapid response of home health resources. It didn't work. You would have thought that we had the superior force, but it was like guerrilla warfare, never knowing where and how scleroderma would strike next.

No time to ask, "why is this happening?" No time for anger. I was just trying to hang on, shell-shocked, in a dazed state. It became my ritual each Monday morning, upon waking, to sit on the edge of the bed, with my head in my hands, thinking about what she couldn't do today that she was able to do the previous Monday.

Our relationship changed. From man and wife, we became patient and caregiver. It became the ultimate high-maintenance relationship. I felt the value of my existence was measured only upon my utilitarian usefulness as a caregiver. It was a spiritual divorce from our previous life, and just as Karen's ID merged with the disease, mine transformed into that of a caregiver.

I had always been the strong one, but now I was afraid to leak even a little of my emotions, for fear it would become an emotional flood that would cause me to loose control, or G-d forbid—cry. If others saw me fall apart, it would shake their confidence; Karen might lose hope, and we would live in a house filled with anarchists. At least that's what I feared. It was a big burden.

We became cut off from the rest of the world; like shut-ins. Visits from friends and family helped break up the monotony, but I began to wonder what they thought we were doing when they weren't there. Good friends, close family were always welcome; acquaintances, long lost relatives were okay, too. FedEx and hospital supply deliveries, Jehovah's Witnesses, and lost strangers could even sometimes be viewed as a welcome break. As visits ended, I envied their ability to close the door and just walk away.

Often, while I walked visitors to the door as they were leaving, they would say something like, "I could never do what you do." I never could graciously take a compliment (I assumed those were compliments). It made me feel uncomfortable. But when people told me I was her savior, courageous, or heroic, to my surprise, it was nice to hear. I didn't really believe it, because my motives were selfish; I just wanted my wife back. But what it did do for me was let me know that other people recognized, at least to some extent, what my life was like.

But I was curious as to why that would be important to me. It wasn't like me. Then I thought of the time right before Karen was diagnosed, when she desperately wanted to know what she had, to confirm that there was really something wrong. I didn't get why it mattered to her so much. To me, you weren't any less sick if a doctor couldn't put a name on it; it just meant that the doctor wasn't smart enough to know. What she needed was validation. The diagnosis helped give her that. And I think that, in a way, validation is what I got when people acknowledged what I was going through.

Chapter 7

PHASE 2

As we endured these months, we were still waiting for the disease to level off and *plateau*. It wasn't happening. We got used to having a continuous medical crisis; it became part of our *normal* routine.

She was getting worse. She stopped believing anyone could help, including me. She could no longer see a future with her getting better; for her, without getting better—she could see no future at all. She lost hope, and began to focus only on what might give her immediate comfort or gratification, even if it was only for a few moments at a time.

I was slow to recognize this change. I was still in the mind-set that it was up to me to save her. It was my job to hang in there while things were tough, decide what was right for her, and wait it out until the disease leveled off, and eventually try to make her better.

With no future in sight, she began to feel that everyone was trying to control her life, especially me: what she ate, when she took her medications, appointment times, what she wore, etc., etc. She couldn't do much on her own, and felt like she had to ask permission for everything; to be moved, to get on the toilet, to brush her teeth.

She resented it, and she was getting increasingly angry. She looked at everything as a win-or-loose situation. If she didn't get what she wanted, it meant someone else must be the winner. I ended up being the enemy, and I helped make myself an excellent target. My bright halo was tarnishing, and the role of caregiver was becoming something less than fulfilling.

I also became increasingly frustrated and angry. She was starting to act like she didn't care about getting better. She continuously made bad choices in what she ate, (with predictable results), and started skipping doses of her medication.

We started arguing, sometimes bitterly, when she began to sporadically resist taking medication and even life-sustaining kidney dialysis. I would go ballistic—I couldn't and wouldn't accept it. I felt that most of my waking hours were devoted just to the care needed to sustain her. Ten percent of that time was spent on looking for, or dreaming about, a new treatment that might help her. That 10 percent was my hope; it motivated me to push on.

Now she was denying me the ability to even maintain consistent care, and I never knew how she would react to a new treatment option. Her resistance destroyed my hope. I felt like all my time and energy had been misappropriated—flushed down the toilet. The frequency and intensity of our arguments were more than we had had in our entire marriage.

For several weeks, maybe more, I was absolutely bewildered as to why she would arbitrarily stop and start medications, express interest in a new treatment and then suddenly drop it. Eventually, I realized she was vacillating between hope and despair. Sometimes the idea of a new treatment gave her a glimmer of hope. Other times, her despair was so deep that she could not dare to think about getting better, for disappointment would be more than she could bear, so she would suddenly drop any new treatment options. And when she thought she was as low as she could go—but kept falling anyway, the thought of skipping medications or treatments was her own version of a nice dream, where she might get lucky and just not have to feel anything anymore.

The more arbitrary she seemed to become in taking medication and treatments, the more generous I became in dispensing large unsolicited doses of anger to anyone that had the misfortune of being nearby, and especially to people that I felt were derailing my efforts. I began to feel irrelevant; I was no longer her savior, just a fixture—caregiving was just a job.

Anybody that I perceived as being a barrier to potentially making her better, or even making her daily care more difficult became road-kill in my path. I was impatient, ill tempered, and rude.

I was most resentful of others when Karen's condition was at its worst. These were the times when my fatigue was greatest and I was emotionally the most fragile. It's when I needed help the most, yet hated to ask; when I did, I felt I was getting mostly talk and little walk. I resented those that I thought (in my own mind) should have known they were not measuring up to what was needed, thus making my life, and in turn, Karen's, more difficult.

I hated what I was becoming. My perceptions had become twisted, and I knew it. I felt like I was racing at 100 miles per hour, with no time to see anything but the fact that time was running out to get her better—and now, because of her resistance, I was actually losing ground.

I started to question why I was doing this, and wondered what the point was. I never considered leaving or just walking out the door, but I began to mellow my attitude towards those who did. Karen and I had a strong marriage; it was hard to imagine a couple surviving this with a weak one.

All Karen seemed to want from me was to be physically close. To sit with her; read next to her; watch TV with her. She didn't see the value of anything else I had to do: not work, not the constant communication with doctors and managed care, or even shopping for food. If I wasn't sitting next to her, she treated it as though I was off enjoying myself.

With everything else I was doing, I felt that just *sitting* with her was a luxury of time I didn't have. Besides, when I did just sit with her, thinking about all that I needed to do put me in an extreme state of agitation, as though I was trapped in a confined space. It was my worst nightmare, like being a prisoner.

And yet, my responsibilities continued to expand— usually by default, or because I didn't feel comfortable asking someone else for help. People marveled at how much I was doing. It was true; I was slowly becoming domesticated (sort of), and learned and understood most of the medical issues that were necessary. But I felt like people had put me on stage, waiting to see my next *impossible* feat. Being recognized for what I was enduring had worked for me in the past, but now it was becoming too heavy of a burden. My *feats* were the only thing in my life that people were noticing—and it was pushing me to the edge of self-destruction.

In the beginning I was more than willing to put my own ambitions on hold. As the disease took its toll and Karen lost hope and only wanted the moments of comfort with me that she could grab, I became totally frustrated. I felt she was trying to sabotage my caregiving efforts and invalidating my personal sacrifices.

I began to think there was something wrong with me. Other people wouldn't allow themselves to be put through this. I almost always trust my instincts, and following them this time felt right at the beginning, but they were obviously leading me astray now. Maybe I was just being stupid. My simple plan to just do the impossible was unraveling: my reduction of work caused us to continuously slide further behind financially; I was often times getting only three to five hours of sleep a day, and was physically on the brink; I had endangered the viability of our family, and now—I felt like I was being forced to watch my wife die. We were imploding. My single-minded determination just seemed to add to everyone's misery.

I would sometimes daydream about finding a way out. Maybe I could just physically run myself into the ground, maybe be lucky enough to end up in the hospital; then I could just shrug, and say, "I tried, but what can I do?" No such luck, I was generally in good health, and considering the circumstances, in excellent condition. Besides, without me, there was no doubt in my mind that

Karen would end up in a nursing home—alone. With the uncertainties of scleroderma, I usually avoided making promises to Karen or the kids; but the one promise I did make to her and myself (and she didn't ask) was that she would never be alone in the care of strangers. No matter how confused, depressed, or desperate I was to find a way out, this one promise I was determined to make non-negotiable—an absolute. It greatly limited my daydreams.

My audio journal helped me tremendously during this time, to sort out emotions—and when that failed, at least made me appear somewhat sane to others. I had been a runner before Karen got sick. For over twenty years it had been a cornerstone in maintaining a good balance between body and soul. Although never a fanatic about it, I had run the Los Angeles Marathon in 1996, motivated mostly by a need to just do it—before I got too old. Now, exhaustion and lack of time eventually put the brakes on my running days.

Karen was not scleroderma's only victim. We were a sad pair—wallowing in self-pity. Karen often said, "I don't want to be me, but I sure don't want to be Mike either." Ditto on that.

PHASE 3

About a year after her diagnosis, Karen was in the hospital—a pretty common event. A week after her admittance for this particular stay, the attending physician, with the usual entourage of five or six residents and medical students, came in for their daily rounds. The faces of the residents and students had become familiar by then, but no one really stood out.

Late that afternoon, one of the residents from that morning came into the room and said he was just visiting. As we talked, his concern and sincerity about how we were doing impressed me. During casual conversation, he made an observation: "For all you are doing for Karen, you're not giving her something she really needs." He didn't elaborate more than to indicate that personal issues were as important as the medical ones. The comment stuck with me.

It didn't cause any sudden realization or epiphany. However, the fact that a resident was able to pick up on this just from what he observed during daily rounds made an impact. I started to think more about my relationship with Karen. I knew that putting all my hopes into the medical side of her care was clearly not working. I began to realize that I had become psychologically detached from her, and she was left feeling emotionally isolated. I began to realize that this had forced both of us to face our emotions alone.

My detachment created a gapping hole in one of the pillars of our marriage—companionship. We had always enjoyed each other's company—just being together. It seemed ironic that by focusing so much on caregiving and medical issues, I was foregoing the opportunity for the one thing I missed most.

Up to this time, I had found it far easier to be her advocate and provide the physical support for caregiving rather than emotional support. It had driven a wedge between us. Maybe I knew I was doing this all along. Perhaps I needed that wedge to help shield me so I wouldn't feel her suffering.

Reconnecting to her emotionally was a slow and painful process. I tried to sit with her more; not be so fidgety; not consider it as a distraction, or jail time. I touched and stroked her just because she liked it, rather than because there was a need to massage or scratch. We started to talk more about our feelings.

It was still hard for me not to hear the clock ticking, thinking that precious time was being diverted from helping her get better. But by this time, anything she allowed me to do was of little value to her; I think she was just humoring me in the least invasive way possible—but it did make me feel like I was at least doing *something*. I never did stop trying, as a caregiver, to make her better. But as her husband, I began to savor our time together and enjoy our resurrected bonds.

She appreciated personal attention that conveyed how much I cared. It was mostly the little stuff. The thing that she loved the most occurred early on in this process when we were looking to buy a recliner for her. I told her I wanted a double recliner so I could be closer to her—her eyes welled with tears. It was the first time in a long time that we were able to look into each other's eyes and see and feel unobstructed love. Even though not much was said afterwards, I heard her on the phone for days, beaming that we got a recliner-for-two because I wanted to sit closer to her.

It was a defining moment for us. Some of our conflicts continued, but from then on, medical care issues seldom superceded our emotional care for each other. Although the symbolism of the dual recliner put us closer together, unfortunately, it didn't overcome her inability to open and raise her arms for a hug.

However, it did allow us emotional intimacy. While we sat on the recliner, my hand was almost always on her. Sometimes late at night, when we were both too tired to start the long ordeal of getting her into bed, we would fall asleep on our recliner, my head on her. Usually, she would never be able to rest comfortably in one position for long, but when we were like that, she seemed to be truly comfortable and at peace.

The other problems didn't go away. We still lived like shut-ins, and I was feeling intellectually starved from lack of outside stimulation (too much Nick at Night). We still argued over what she was eating and what pills to take, but the volume became more muted.

This renewed closeness came at a price. I began to feel her suffering. I never had much use for sympathy—it seemed too gratuitous and contained too many empty words for me. What did come out of me though (and until then was never sure that it was in me) was a profound depth of compassion and empathy. So much so, that at times, her suffering became mine. I would sometimes even dream that I had become her, enduring what she endured. Other times I thought in parables, thinking about what it would be like to be her: maybe being put in a straight-jacket, sitting in an airline seat (coach of course), taxiing down the runway, unable to stand up; my knees jammed into the seat in front of me; people's bodies overlapping their seats onto me; condemned to taxi forever—never to take-off, but also never to stop and walk on earth again.

Though the emotional price was high, I rededicated myself to bringing Karen the moments of pleasure she craved. I found it impossible to deny her anything I thought would make her happy.

She took great pleasure from anything that she saw as a sign of my caring. Most of it involved her grooming. Fortunately, I was not judged on my proficiency, only on my effort. Others could do better, but it didn't matter. Even when I used her lip liner as eyeliner, I could do no wrong. She would proudly display the pedicure I gave her to the nurses at the dialysis center, even though it was difficult to distinguish where one nail ended and the next began. It took awhile, but actually (I don't want to brag) I really did get pretty good at all this stuff.

The kitchen had always been her turf. She had been a great cook and entertainer. She loved and treasured her kitchen, and it represented one of the many important things she lost to scleroderma. It was extremely difficult for her to watch the kids and me using a favorite pot, or a delicate plate. She wanted us to take as good a care of her things as she did. It was an impossible task, but we tried.

I wasn't much of a cook, and my tastes had moved away from Karen's rich cooking style over the years. I wanted to please her though, and was determined to learn to cook the way she wanted, even though it was usually a symbolic effort, because what food she did eat hardly ever stayed down.

I knew that I was really getting into it, when one day, while reading a post in a scleroderma digest on the Internet, someone was giving the details of what looked like a great soup recipe—a quick cut and paste and I gave it a try. It gave Karen great pleasure as I attempted to make her what she would like. I became her hands and legs in the kitchen, following her instructions. It got to a point where she not only appreciated my effort, but eventually seemed to actually like what I made for her.

None of our daughters cooked (I never noticed this fact until Karen got sick) but the youngest one at least had an interest in it. She became Karen's apprentice. One Thanksgiving, under Karen's direction, she made all of our favorites; it was a highlight for everyone. Today, our daughter has graduated to keeper of the family recipes.

I mentioned before that we lived like shut-ins. Actually, that wasn't completely true. It was just that most of the time when we left the house, it was for a doctor's appointment or dialysis. We weren't able to get out as often as we liked, just to do normal things—we felt encumbered by the disease. Scleroderma followed us to stores, theatres, and restaurants. Often times it just wasn't worth the trouble.

Parking was always a problem. With all the laws I heard about, I just assumed that we could get handicapped access most everywhere. But many times, there just weren't any open spaces. We often parked at the end of the parking lot in 100-degree heat, or when it was raining. Many of the people we wheeled by as they got into their handicapped spaces appeared to have no physical disability.

I know that this is an unfair judgment. I know you can't always see someone's disability. Some could even be other scleroderma patients who have the added burden of having their disability hidden. Beyond that though, my experience makes me think that there is a general abuse by people using placards who are not disabled and who hide behind the presumption of having a hidden disability. I feel that the lack of respect and enforcement for disabled parking makes life tougher for everyone, especially for those with a *hidden* disability. In any case, the lack of handicapped parking was a factor as to why we were shut-in as much as we were.

Even if we were able to get from the parking lot into the store, finding, and being able to get into bathrooms was another hurdle. I felt very uncomfortable because I had to go into the ladies room with Karen so I could lift her on and off the wheelchair. I hated it, even though some of my new bathroom mates tried to make me feel more comfortable, pleasantly smiling, even offering help. Sometimes women even struck up conversations. It only made me move faster.

One of our truly great pleasures was to take a long drive in the car. Access did dictate where we stopped for food and bathrooms, but our goal was mostly just to drive, with no particular destination in mind. It was like being able to run away from our scleroderma-infested environment and just talk. We talked mostly about what was good in our lives; we expressed our appreciation for what we had, and especially for each other. It was also a time when we each freely expressed what we hated most about scleroderma.

Karen used to be very intuitive, and was almost psychic in being able to read my thoughts. When we used to play knowledge games with others, and were on opposing teams, I felt like she could reach into my brain for the answers I knew she didn't know; I accused her of cheating. That didn't happen too much after she got sick; I think scleroderma just got in the way. Sometimes our drives were a bust and we would have to go back home if she suddenly got sick; but mostly, it was a time for sharpening our focus on each other.

Our problems never went away, but more important things could overshadow them. We had banded together, in the same foxhole, and usually became allies rather than competitors against a common foe. It helped to create a deeper relationship than ever before.

Karen also acquired a new appreciation for nature: she would ask me to pull over to interrupt a drive on the coast highway, and even though she was still cold in the warmth of summer, would ask to have her window rolled down so she could turn her face to the ocean and feel and taste the salty air. If she saw a baby lizard sunning itself on a hot rock, she would say, "that's what I want to be." When a family of jackrabbits moved into our yard, she would spend half an afternoon outside the front door, waiting to see a baby one streak by.

Scleroderma permanently changed me. In the beginning, I arrogantly thought I could enforce my will and control the disease; I almost sacrificed everything and everybody in the process. Scleroderma made me much more aware of other people's suffering and I learned more about myself than I thought possible. In the end, the power of the disease left me humble.

Karen and I couldn't change what scleroderma did to her physically, but we did choose to learn to live in spite of the disease, as best we could, and enjoy what we had.

Even having to witness all her suffering, I am grateful for this time. The little moments of pleasure that she so desperately craved became the sweetest of moments in my life, in what was, at its best, the most bittersweet of times.

Epilogue

This page was an afterthought. Initially, it was my intent to let my personal account speak for itself. As I noted at the beginning of Chapter 7, I wasn't going to give you a checklist of what to do. Besides, if I had some sort of life-altering advice, I'd just tell you.

Even though I don't have a checklist, I would like to leave you with how I look back on all of this. It's not really that much different than before—just clearer and more obvious.

Some of the experiences, no matter how hard I try, I will never be able to forget—but mostly, I think about the memories that I savor, that will always be with me. I don't beat myself up about the things I learned the hard way. I have few regrets. We were inexperienced and unprepared to deal with such a catastrophe; we did the best we could under the circumstances.

But I do think about all the problems caused by my unwillingness to accept anything less than *getting her better*. It destroyed our ability to communicate; emotionally, it prevented us from openly sharing our feelings, and in practical terms, stopped us from talking about what was *do-able*. It prevented me from having any kind of a backup plan—when things went wrong, my only alternative was to increase my effort—scleroderma devoured me.

In the end, we were lucky—obviously not in a traditional sense. But we were lucky to have eventually recognized how much we missed each other—and to do something about it: we changed the way we communicated. Our old system of intuition and coded words proved to be useless in confronting scleroderma. Our new system was simply based on our emotional care of each other; it laid the groundwork that saved and resurrected what we both valued the most.

As for Karen, I will always be grateful to her for giving me the missing pieces of my life. She was always smart, and always true to herself. Luckily for me, she never lost sight of what she valued the most; it was my greatest fortune to have been the centerpiece of her life.

APPENDIX A

Scleroderma Press is interested in publishing profiles of scleroderma patients and their caregivers. If you are interested in participating, please send us a letter that answers the following questions, or, e-mail us.

- Year of diagnosis

- Age

- Brief description of disease involvements

- Do you currently work?

- Do you have children living with you?

- Is a family member your caregiver?

- If yes, primary responsibilities of caregiver.

Please send us a letter with the above information to:
Scleroderma Press
P.O. Box 261671
Encino, CA 91426-1671

Or e-mail us: SclerodermaPress@aol.com

Please make sure to include your address, phone number, and e-mail address.

APPENDIX B—Additional Resources

The Megasite Project: A comprehensive site that evaluates various features, such as frequency of updates, peer-reviewed, and even notes if the site uses cookies. Most of it is focused on professionals, but also has a lot of information that scleroderma patients can use. Take the time to browse this site; the resources noted contain some of the best sites for health information. This site is a project of medical librarians. http://www.lib.umich.edu/megasite/toc.html

Healthfinder: The government's gateway site to health information. http://www.healthfinder.gov

RxList: An Internet drug and alternative medicine reference www.rxlist.com

Pharma-Lexicon: A medical and pharmaceutical abbreviations dictionary. http://www.pharma-lexicon.com

FDA: Site warns of the risks of buying prescription drugs online. www.fda.gov/oc/buyonline/default.htm

The National Association of Boards of Pharmacy (NABP)
Established certification of standards for online pharmacies. www.nabp.net/vipps/consumer/listall.asp

The United States Pharmacopoeia: Establishes standards to ensure the quality of medicines for human use. This organization is also starting a pilot program that will standardize herbs and other dietary supplements. www.usp.org

CONSUMER HEALTH SITES

CBShealthwatch: www.cbshealthwatch.com

Consumer Reports on Health: www.consumerreports.ort/services/health.html

HealthAtoZ: http://www.healthatoz.com/

InteliHealth: http://www.intelihealth.com

Mayo Clinic Health Oasis: www.mayohealth.org

Medscape: A commercial medical information site for the consumers and professionals. http://www.medscape.com/

WebMD: www.webmd.com

FOOTNOTES

Many of the references in this book are Internet links. The web is a huge advantage for the reader, in being able to go directly to these sites for additional information. Unfortunately, the downside is, that over a period of time, some of these links may be deleted by the host-site.

---

[1] The Scleroderma Book: A Guide for Patients and Families. Maureen D. Mayes, MD. Oxford University Press 1999

[2] Systemic Sclerosis, Philip J. Clements (Editor), Daniel E. Furst (Editor), Lippincott, Williams & Wilkins, 1996

[3] "Lawmaker focuses on Scleroderma", The Tulsa World, March 27, 2000

[4] The Grand Rapids Press; Feb 19, 2001

[5] Orphan Drug Act of 1983. Food and Drug Administration Office of Orphan Product Development http://www.fda.gov/orphan/index.htm

[6] "Handout on Health- Scleroderma." The National Institute of Health Clearinghouse, 1 AMS Circle, Bethesda, MD 20892-3675. http://www.niams.nih.gov/hi/topics/scleroderma/scleroderma.htm

[7] National Institute of Arthritis and Musculoskeletal and Skin Diseases, Information Clearinghouse, National Institutes of Health, 1 AMS Circle, Bethesda, Maryland 20892-3675. Phone: (301) 495-4484 or (877) 22-NIAMS (toll free). TTY: (301) 565-2966

[8] NIAMS press release- http://www.niams.nih.gov/ne/ press/2001/06_22.htm. New contact information, effective Feb. 18, 2002: Scleroderma Family Registry and DNA Repository, University of Texas Health Science Center at Houston, 6431 Fannin, MSB 5.270, Houston, TX 77030. (800) 736-6864, Fax: (713)500-0580. Registry Coordinator: Marilyn Perry.

[9] Handout on Health- Scleroderma. The National Institute of Health Clearinghouse, 1 AMS Circle, Bethesda, MD 20892-3675. http://www.niams.nih.gov/hi/topics/scleroderma/scleroderma.htm

[10] Scleroderma Research Foundation. 2320 Bath Street #315, Santa Barbara, CA 93105. (805)563-9133. www.srfcure.org

[11] Scleroderma Foundation. 12 Kent Way, Suite 101, Byfield, MA 01922. (800)722-4673. http://www.scleroderma.org/

[12] Computer Retrieval of Information on Scientific Projects. https://www-commons.cit.nih.gov/crisp/. Keyword: scleroderma.

[13] Scleroderma Clinical Trials Consortium (SCTC) http://www.sctc-online.org/

[14] American Autoimmune Related Diseases Association. 22100 Gratiot Ave., E. Detroit, MI 48021. (586)776-3900. http://www.aarda.org/

[15] Cooperative Study Group For Autoimmune Disease Prevention, September 7, 2000. http://grants.nih.gov/grants/guide/rfa-files/RFA-AI-00-016.html

[16] Press release, American Autoimmune Related Diseases Association, September 28, 2000. http://www.aarda.org/press_release10.html

[17] "New Legislation Creates Landmark Autoimmune Diseases Committee at NIH", PR Newswire, 09/28/2000

[18] Centers for Disease Control and Prevention. 800-311-3435. http://www.cdc.gov/

[19] Food and Drug Administration (FDA). 5600 Fishers Lane, Rockville MD 20857-0001. 888-463-6332. http://www.fda.gov/

[20] Scleroderma Voice, Winter 2001-2002.

[21] SCOR- The first Specialized Center of Research in scleroderma was established in December 1997, through a NIAMS grant for $3.5 million for 4 years, and includes support from the NIH Office of Research on Women's Health. http://www.nih.gov/news/pr/dec97/niams-15.htm

[22] "Handout on Health- Scleroderma." NIH Clearinghouse, 1 AMS Circle, Bethesda, MD 20892-3675. http://www.niams.nih.gov/hi/topics/scleroderma/scleroderma.htm

[23] "A Mother And Child Union: Trading Cells", The Boston Globe, May 8, 2001

[24] Medline, June 2001.
http://www.ncbi.nlm.nih.gov/PubMed

[25] Scleroderma Clinical Trials Consortium Lung Study.
http://sclerodermalungstudy.medsch.ucla.edu

[26] Medline, Dec. 2000/ The Th1/Th2 paradigm in the pathogenesis of scleroderma, and its modulation by thalidomide.
http://www.ncbi.nlm.nih.gov/PubMed

[27] "Could this end the misery of freezing hands for millions?" Daily Mail, UK- 10/09/2001.

[28] Raynaud's & Scleroderma Association. 112 Crewe Road, Alsager, Cheshire ST7 2JA (UK). Telephone 44 (0)1270 872776 Fax 44 (0)1270 883556. http://www.raynauds.demon.co.uk/

[29] NIH database of clinical trials. http://clinicaltrials.gov/

[30] "Data Presented at Third International Conference on Relaxin", PR Newswire; New York; Oct 26, 2000

[31] "How to talk to your doctor." *Morning Call*; Allentown; Jun 20, 1999.

[32] Scleroderma Foundation. (800)-722-4673. http://www.scleroderma.org/support.html

[33] Scleroderma Research Foundation. (805)563-9133. www.srfcure.org Scleroderma Foundation. (800)722-4673. http://www.scleroderma.org/ Scleroderma Clinical Trials Consortium (SCTC) http://www.sctc-online.org/

[34] Search Medline. Keywords: scleroderma AND [city/state]. http://www.ncbi.nlm.nih.gov

[35] American College of Rheumatology. 1800 Century Place, Suite 250, Atlanta, GA 30345. (404) 633-3777; fax: (404) 633-1870. http://www.rheumatology.org/

[36] American Medical Association.. 515 N. State Street, Chicago, Illinois, 60610. 312-464-5000. http://www.ama-assn.org/

[37] American Board Of Medical Specialty. 1007 Church Street, Suite 404, Evanston, IL 60201-5913. Phone verification (866) ASK-ABMS. Phone: (847) 491-9091 | Fax: (847) 328-3596. http://www.abms.org/

[38] Association of State Medical Board Executive Directors. http://www.docboard.org

[39] American College of Rheumatology, 1800 Century Place, Suite 250, Atlanta, GA 30345. (404) 633-3777; fax: (404) 633-1870. http://www.rheumatology.org/

[40] Public Citizen Health Research Group. (202) 588-1000. http://www.citizen.org/hrg/ & http://www.citizen.org/HRG/ QDSITE/QDHOMEPAGE/QDHOMEPAGE/qdhome.html

[41] Scleroderma Press, P.O. Box 261671, Encino, CA 91426-1671. Voice & fax: (818) 708-0487. $17 per PMO. www.SclerodermPress.com

[42] American Medical Consumers. 818/957-3508. Basic membership pack $155. www.medconsumer.com/

[43] CapMed, P.O. Box 18846, Huntsville, AL 35804. (256) 881-6030. $49.95. http://capmed.com/

[44] Freeware/Shareware. Use key word "medical, personal medical records" etc. www.download.com & www.tucows.com

[45] www.SclerodermaPress.com

[46] Pharmaceutical Research and Manufacturers of America (PhRMA) (800) 762-4636. www.phrma.org.

[47] Policy Almanac. Managed Care Issues. http://www.policyalmanac.org/health/hmos.shtml#Related%20Sites

[48] U.S. News & World Report HMO ratings (many other useful surveys too). http://www.norc.uchicago.edu/studies/homepage.htm & http://www.norc.uchicago.edu/studies/health.htm#hmos

[49] National Opinion Research Center. 1155 East 60th Street, Chicago, IL 60637. (773) 256-6000. http://www.norc.uchicago.edu/

[50] National Committee for Quality Assurance - 2000 L Street NW Suite 500 - Washington, DC 20036 - (202) 955-3500. http://hprc.ncqa.org/

[51] Accreditation Association for Ambulatory Health Care, Inc., AAAHC. 9933 Lawler Avenue, Suite 460, Skokie, IL 60077. (847) 676-9610 http://www.aaahc.org/

[52] Joint Commission on Accreditation of Healthcare Organizations. One Renaissance Blvd. Oakbrook Terrace, IL 60181. http://www.jcaho.org

[53] American Accreditation HealthCare Commission. 1275 K Street NW, Suite 1100 | Washington, DC 20005, 202-216-9010. http://www.urac.org

[54] Standard and Poors. http://www.standardandpoors.com & http://www.standardandpoors.com/RatingsActions/RatingsLists/Insurance/InsuranceStrengthRatings.html

[55] A.M. Best financial ratings- insurance companies http://www.ambest.com

[56] Moodys financial ratings- insurance companies www.moodys.com

[57] Weiss Ratings- financial ratings- insurance companies. http://www.weissratings.com

[58] "A Referee in Disputes Between Patients, HMOs", Los Angeles Times, July 30, 2001.

[59] Each state is different. Check with the HMO providers in your home state for availability of senior coverage.

[60] Medicare customer service: 800-633-4227. http://www.medicare.gov/

[61] Journal of Financial Planning; Oct. 2001. GAO review of Medigap insurance.

[62] Remember, Medicaid is called by a different name in each state. Contact your home state office. General information can be obtained at the federal site: http://www.hcfa.gov/medicaid/medicaid.htm

[63] National Center for Policy Analysis. Medical Savings Accounts overview. http://www.hmopage.org/msawhat.html

[64] American Council of Life Insurers. 1001 Pennsylvania Avenue, N.W. Washington, D.C. 20004. http://www.acli.com/

[65] U.S. Department of Housing and Urban Development. Annual Report on foreclosures, 2000. 451 7th Street S.W., Washington, DC 20410. (202) 708-1112   TTY: (202) 708-1455. http://www.hud.gov

[66] Disability Report Form Guide. 800-772-1213 http://www.ssa.gov/disability/3368/

[67] Social Security-Disability http://www.ssa.gov/OP_Home/rulings/di-toc.html

[68] Social Security-SSI. 800-772-1213. http://www.ssa.gov/pubs/11000.html

[69] U.S. Department of Labor, Pension and Welfare Benefits Administration, 200 Constitution Avenue, NW Washington, DC 20210-1111. (202)693-8300. http://askpwba.dol.gov/

[70] Internal Revenue Service. (800)829-1040 http://www.irs.gov/

[71] CORBA http://www.dol.gov/dol/pwba/public/pubs/cobrafs.htm

[72] The Health Insurance Portability and Accountability Act of 1996 (HIPAA) http://www.hcfa.gov/hipaa/hipaahm.htm

[73] Agency for Healthcare Research & Quality, Office of Health Care Information, Suite 501, Executive Office Center, 2101 East Jefferson Street, Rockville, MD 20852 http://www.ahrq.gov/research/ltcix.htm

[74] National Home Care Council. 202/547-6586

[75] National Association for Home Care 202/547-7424 or 800/677-1116

[76] Health Insurance Association of America-Long term care. 1201 F Street N.W., Suite 500, Washington, D.C. 20004-1204, (202) 824-1600. http://www.hiaa.org/cons/guideltc.html

[77] Joint Commission On Accreditation Of Health Care Organization. (630) 916-5600

[78] Patient Self Determination Act http://archfami.ama-assn.org/issues/v7n5/abs/foc7036.html

[79] Partnership For Caring. 800-989-9455.
http://www.partnershipforcaring.org/HomePage

[80] Policy Almanac. http://www.policyalmanac.org/health/hmos.shtml,
and Afro - American Red Star; Washington, D.C.; Apr 21, 2001.
"Medical privacy regulation to go into effect"

[81] Plasmaphoresis removes certain components from a blood cell,
including antibodies, with the hope of getting the immune system back
into sync.

[82] The National Association for Chiropractic Medicine (NACM). 15427
Baybrook Drive. Houston, TX 77062. (281)280-8262.
http://www.chiromed.org/.

[83] American Assoc. of Acupuncture and Oriental Medicine. 433 Front
St. Catasauqua, PA 18032. (888) 500-7999. http://www.aaom.org/

[84] http://www.acupuncture.com. For your information only. (This site is
for marketing purposes.)

[85] FDA website. "Homeopathy: Real Medicine or Empty Promises?"
http://www.fda.gov/fdac/features/096_home.html

[86] National Institute of Homeopathy. For your information only. (This
is not an authoritative site). http://www.netguruindia.com/oncampus/
oncampus_cal/nih/nih_index.htm

[87] The American Association of Naturopathic Physicians. 8201
Greensboro Drive, Suite 300, McLean, VA 22102. (703) 610-9037.
http://www.naturopathic.org/

[88] The National Association for Holistic Aromatherapy. 4509 Interlake
Ave N., #233, Seattle, WA 98103-6773. (888)ASK-NAHA .
http://www.naha.org/

[89] American Demographics Magazine. Survey, January 2001.

[90] Employee Benefit Plan Review, May 1999.

[91] HerbMed® An interactive, electronic herbal database – provides
hyperlinked access to the scientific data underlying the use of herbs for
health. It is an evidence-based information resource for professionals,
researchers, and the general public. http://www.herbmed.org/

[92] http://www.ncbi.nlm.nih.gov/PubMed

[93] Center for Evidence-Based Practice, State University of New York-
EBM. http://www.upstate.edu/fmed/cebp/

[94] National Summit on Patient Safety Data Collection and Use
http://www.ahcpr.gov/qual/taskforce/psagenda.htm

[95] New England Journal of Medicine http://content.nejm.org/.

[96] Business Wire; New York; Oct 19, 2000. IMS HEALTH Reports, U.S. Pharmaceutical Promotional Spending

[97] "The Influence of Drug Companies on Clinical Trials", Wall Street Journal, September 10, 2001.

[98] Wall Street Journal, June 22, 2001

[99] PubMed- May 2001. Placebo report. http://www.ncbi.nlm.nih.gov/PubMed

[100] Pharmaceutical Executive, January 2000.

[101] The Alternative Medicine Foundation. http://www.amfoundation.org/

[102] The Arthritis Foundation's Guide to Alternative Therapies, by Judith Horstman, William J. Arnold (Editor), The Arthritis Foundation, 1999. available through bookstores, or directly from the Arthritis Foundation. (800)283-7800; http://www.arthritis.org/

[103] The White House Commission on Complementary and Alternative Medicine Policy. 6707 Democracy Boulevard, Room 880, MS – 5467, Bethesda, Maryland 20892. (301) 435-7592. www.whccamp.hhs.gov.

[104] National Center for Complementary and Alternative Medicine, NCCAM Clearinghouse, P.O. Box 7923, Gaithersburg, Maryland 20898. (888)-644-6226, http://nccam.nih.gov/

[105] http://www.chinausahealthcare.org./

[106] Rand Study on getting health information from the Internet. http://ehealth.chcf.org/view.cfm?section=Industry&itemID=3973

[107] URAC Health Web Site Accreditation Program. www.urac.org

[108] List of accredited sites and those in progress of accreditation. http://www.urac.org/news/releases/011212hwsaccreditations.htm

[109] Pew Internet & American Life. 2000 report –"Internet & Health"

[110] The Lancet Publishing Group, 84 Theobald's Road, London, WC1X 8RR, UK http://www.thelancet.com/

[111] http://www.quackwatch.com/

[112] Typical Search Engines: www.yahoo.com, www.Excite.com, www.AltaVista.com, www.Hotbot.com.

[113] "What are meta search engines?" UC Berkeley Library: www.lib.berkeley.edu/TeachingLib/Guides/Internet/MetaSearch.html

[114] Internet Public Library www.ipl.org/ref.

[115] Librarians' Index to the Internet
http://sunsite.berkeley.edu/internetindex

[116] World Wide Web Virtual Library. http://vlig.org

[117] Tracking federal legislation/Thomas
http://thomas.loc.gov/ . You can also get to this site by cruising through
the Library of Congress: www.lcweb.loc.gov

[118] Library of Congress. http://www.loc.gov/

[119] PubMed www.ncbi.nlm.nih.gov/PubMed

[120] Newsgroups can be found all over the web. An example of a
newsgroup: go to www.Google.com. Click on "groups". For the
scleroderma support group, search "scleroderma". For information on
participating in this group, click on "Post a new message to
alt.support.scleroderma".

[121] Examples of mailing lists:
http://groups.yahoo.com/group/sdandasupport/
http://groups.yahoo.com/group/sdworld/ and

[122] Caregiver stories: Saving Milly: Love, Politics, and Parkinson's
Disease. Morton Kondracke, PublicAffairs, 2001, NY. Surviving Your
Spouse's Chronic Illness: A Compassionate Guide. Chris McGonigle,
PhD., An Owl Book, Henry Holt & Co. New York, 1999.

[123] National Family Caregivers Association. (800)896-3650, fax
(301)942-2302. www.NFCACARES.ORG

About Karen . . .

Karen was a life-long volunteer and fundraiser for many charities. Neither she nor any of her family or friends had any of the diseases represented by these charities. She was involved because, as she would often say, it enriched her life.

Thus for Karen, it became important to involve as many people as possible in supporting a charity. Because of her, there are hundreds of people today that continue their charitable involvement.

Just before her death, she created The Karen Brown Scleroderma Foundation. It is the goal of the Foundation to involve many of the people whose lives she touched, and to instill her spirit in a new generation of volunteers to raise money for scleroderma research.

It was her desire not to seek the support of scleroderma patients and families. She wanted to create new money for scleroderma research. If you would like to know more about Karen, please visit the Foundation's website at:

www.KBSfoundation.org

Personal Medical Organizer

For information, visit the Scleroderma Press website at

www.SclerodermaPress.com